Introduction to Medical Radiographic Imaging

Compiled, edited, and written in part by:

Robert J. Pizzutiello, Jr., M.S.
and
John E. Cullinan, R.T. (R)

for
Eastman Kodak Company

Health Sciences Division
EASTMAN KODAK COMPANY
Rochester, New York 14650

Front cover chest radiograph courtesy of
R. J. Chambers, M.D., Ottawa Civic Hospital, Ottawa, Ontario, Canada

Library of Congress Catalog Number: 93-72374

ISBN: 0-8798-0485
© Eastman Kodak Company, 1993
Printed in the United States of America

Printed on recycled paper containing 10% post-consumer waste fiber, using soy-based inks.

Foreword

The first edition of a booklet on the principles of radiography was published by Eastman Kodak Company in 1918. The manual was entitled *X-rays* and was the forerunner of *The Fundamentals of Radiography*. Over the years, 12 editions of *X-rays* were published. The title was changed to *X-rays in Medicine* in 1930 and to *Eastman X-ray Laboratory Manual* in 1934. The first edition of *The Fundamentals of Radiography* was published in 1938, with its 12th edition published in 1980. *Introduction to Medical Radiographic Imaging* preserves the core of the 12th Edition and adds information on current technology. Some materials in this text are new, other materials are derived or reproduced from technical articles published by Eastman Kodak Company. *Introduction to Medical Radiographic Imaging* is part of Kodak's ongoing support to the field of medical radiographic imaging.

Biographical Sketches

Robert J. Pizzutiello, Jr.

Bob received his M.S.E.E. from the University of Rochester, Rochester, New York in 1978. He began teaching diagnostic radiology residents and radiologic technologists in 1979. In 1983, he was certified by the American Board of Radiology in Therapeutic Radiological Physics. In 1993, Bob was certified in Diagnostic Imaging Physics by the American Board of Medical Physics. Currently, he is president of Upstate Medical Physics, Inc., where he practices diagnostic imaging physics for hospitals and clinics.

John E. Cullinan

Jack was registered with the American Registry of Radiologic Technologists in 1951. After a tour of duty in the United States Navy, he worked for many years with hospitals in the Commonwealth of Pennsylvania. In 1968, he was elected a Fellow in the American Society of Radiologic Technologists. In 1973, Jack joined Eastman Kodak Company as a senior technical associate. Jack retired from Eastman Kodak Company in 1991.

Acknowledgments

Eastman Kodak Company would like to extend recognition and gratitude to several people. A special thanks goes to Dr. Joel E. Gray, Professor of Radiologic Physics at Mayo Clinic, Rochester, Minnesota for his invaluable review of the entire manuscript. The academic and educational viewpoints were reviewed and enhanced by the following people: Peter Blacher, Professor and Department Head, Radiologic Technology, Erie Community College, Buffalo, New York, and Lynne Freeland, Director of Education, St. James Mercy Hospital, School of Radiography, Hornell, New York. David Stornelli also provided a valuable perspective as a medical student at the University of Rochester, School of Medicine, Rochester, New York.

Sincere appreciation is extended for the support and contributions of numerous people at Eastman Kodak Company, Health Sciences Division, Rochester, New York. In particular, to Arthur G. Haus for his continuous project support, his assistance in determining the scope of this text, for providing material for the book, and for coordinating the technical contributions and reviews.

The following people at Eastman Kodak Company reviewed and provided helpful comments on the manuscript: Adrienne Berend, Dr. Phillip C. Bunch, Donald L. Burrows, Robert E. Dickerson, Judy M. Giambrone-Pribe, Richard S. Hirschland, Susan M. Jaskulski, Douglas E. Pfeiffer, Stephen J. Pflanz, Linda J. Roach, Thomas F. Rose, Eric E. Sumner, Dr. Bruce R. Whiting, William D. Whitmore, Timothy J. Wojcik, and Roseann K. Jackura, Project Coordinator. Kodak also extends its appreciation to David A. Smith for his continuing support of this project.

Eastman Kodak also thanks the following people for their dedication to quality and timeliness in the planning and preparation of this text: Lorraine Trude, Editorial Services and Thomas E. Cone, Art Director and Designer, Pierce Brown Associates Inc.; M. Doris DeFreze, Support Services, The Communications Shop; and Victoria L. Frederic, Administrative Assistant, Upstate Medical Physics, Inc.

Preface

This volume is intended for the student of medical radiographic imaging. It has been written to meet the practical and educational needs of student radiographers, resident radiologists, medical students, medical physics students, as well as other health care professionals.

In the modern health care environment, it would be difficult to imagine much of what we do in patient care without the contribution of medical radiographic imaging. Therefore, this text serves as an introduction for all health care professionals who require a better understanding of this subject matter. It is our hope that physicians, nurses, physician assistants, medical assistants, and other health care professionals will also find useful material in this book.

Conventions

References are listed in detail at the end of the text. Each reference is identified with a superscript number, such as [1]. All references to articles, books and standards are numbered chronologically in order of first appearance from the beginning to the end of the text. Most, but not all, references are cited within figure captions or legends.

Important terms appear in boldface type when first introduced and defined. Other terms are italicized either when first introduced, but not yet defined, or for emphasis.

Contents

Introduction

In 1895, the first medical radiographs intrigued the medical and scientific community. Those early, crude images were made using invisible rays to demonstrate structures equally invisible to the human eye. Stimulated by those early images, an entire "technology" has evolved. Members of the scientific, medical, and manufacturing community have forged a cooperative alliance based on a common, unifying purpose: To produce quality medical radiographic images at dose levels that are As Low As Reasonably Achievable (ALARA) for the betterment of patient care.

This volume explores the origin and nature of x rays and how they are used to produce medical radiographic images. The book focuses on the concepts that govern the production of high-quality images through the use of radiographic film and intensifying screens. While modern medical imaging technology extends beyond these modalities, screen-film imaging and film-based image storage will continue to be the backbone of medical imaging for the foreseeable future. Furthermore, the concepts and techniques discussed in this volume form the foundation of imaging knowledge and are the basis upon which all other imaging methods are built.

If we better understand the physical principles behind the radiographs we see on the viewbox, we will learn that imaging every anatomical segment—whether it be chest, bone or breast—presents its own set of technical requirements and difficulties. In addition, we must never forget that each patient is a living, breathing human being with a different body shape, size, and composition. In our dual capacity as care-giver and imaging specialist, we must adapt our techniques to provide the best, most appropriate images for the person on whom we focus our attention. For this reason, conceptual presentations in this text are followed by sample radiographs wherever possible.

As in all academic endeavors, the more we know, the more we realize how much more there is to learn. No simple solutions exist to the problems presented by our efforts to achieve quality medical radiographic images. As we better understand all of the physical principles that control image formation, we realize that creating the "perfect" image is a practical impossibility. The nature of imaging techniques and products requires the educated user to understand the compromises involved in producing an image and to make judicious choices to achieve his or her goals. For example, we will learn that when a high-contrast image is desirable, some sacrifice in latitude or patient dose is required.

We must also avoid the temptation to look for the "ideal" product to solve our imaging problems. Rather, we must look upon the available imaging products as a menu of technical choices, with each selection designed to meet a particular imaging need. The purpose of this volume is to prepare the imaging specialist to make intelligent judgments that result in the highest quality images possible with the least amount of exposure to our patients.

Chapter 1

X rays and Their Production

The radiograph is perhaps the most fundamental element of diagnostic medical imaging. The image we see on a viewbox is the result of a complex series of physical phenomena and interactions. X rays are produced in the target of an x-ray tube and interact with everything in their path between the tube and the x-ray film. Once the x rays encounter the body of the patient, some will penetrate the patient and some will not. The radiographic image is made from the x rays that penetrate the patient and ultimately produce blackening of the x-ray film. Those x rays that do not emerge from the patient, but are absorbed (attenuated), also contribute to the image. In a sense, these x rays are "conspicuous by their absence"— since they do not darken the film, they contribute to lighter areas on the film.

If radiology were as simple as black and white, it would be a trivial specialty at best. Many factors, however, affect the way in which a particular anatomical site will appear on an image. A **radiograph** is a flat, two-dimensional representation of interactions that occur in a three-dimensional subject, that is, the patient. To complicate the situation further, the shades of gray in a radiograph are produced as a result of other occurrences between the x-ray target and the film, not just those resulting from patient anatomy. For example, clothing, jewelry, orthopedic casts, and radiographic or processing artifacts also affect the diagnostic quality of the radiograph. A high-quality image is one in which the amount of anatomical information in the image is maximized, while distractions are minimized.

Let's begin by investigating the source of our image—the x-ray beam.

WHAT ARE X RAYS?

X rays are a form of electromagnetic radiation. The word **radiation** means *transfer of energy*. Electromagnetic radiation or energy has the following characteristics.

1. The energy can travel in a vacuum. This is different from sound energy, which requires a medium such as water or tissue to travel.

2. The energy travels at what we commonly call the *speed of light* (about 186,000 miles/sec. [3×10^8 m/sec.] in a vacuum).

3. The energy is quantized, that is, it can exist only in fixed, discrete levels, rather than over a continuous range. Most important for imaging purposes is the energy of the **quanta**, which determines their properties in interacting with patients, intensifying screens, x-ray film or other objects.

It is difficult to imagine what an x ray looks like. We can neither see a quantum of energy, nor can we easily comprehend the transfer of energy at the speed of light. In order to assist the thought process, a scientific model is frequently used. A good model has two purposes: to provide us with a mental image that we can relate to, and to help us to accurately predict the behavior of a given phenomenon.

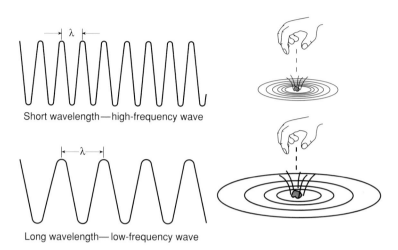

Short wavelength—high-frequency wave

Long wavelength— low-frequency wave

Figure 1–1 Wavelength Comparison. The lambda (λ) symbol is used to identify the distance in a short wavelength (high-frequency) wave (top left) versus a long wavelength (low-frequency) wave (bottom left). These waves can be equated to dropping pebbles into a pond. A small pebble creates waves of a short wavelength; a larger rock creates longer wavelength waves.

Sometimes a single model proves to be inadequate in meeting our requirements. With x rays (as with all electromagnetic radiation), both the "wave" and the "particle" models are used. That is, at times, it serves our needs to consider electromagnetic radiation as a **particle**, or **photon**. A photon is a discrete bundle of energy having no mass, which meets the three characteristics described earlier. You might think of an infinitesimally small bullet being shot from a gun. The energy of such a bullet might be thought of as its speed—the higher the speed (kinetic energy), the higher its energy. Remember, of course, that all photons travel at essentially the same speed—the speed of light.

At other times, our needs are better met by using a **wave** as a model of electromagnetic radiation, which is composed of undulating electric and magnetic fields. Consider the wave pattern that is produced when a pebble is tossed into a still pond. The energy of the pebble is converted into water waves. The wavelength of these water waves is the distance from crest to crest, or trough to trough **(Figure 1–1)**. In an electromagnetic wave, the energy, E, of the wave is related to the wavelength, λ, by this simple formula:

$$E = h \, c / \lambda$$

where c is the speed of light and h is a constant, known as Planck's constant. Since energy and wavelength are inversely proportional, shorter wavelengths correspond to higher energy and longer wavelengths correspond to lower energy.

In either model, each photon or wave of radiation can travel through a vacuum at the speed of light. Most important, each photon or wave has a specific energy that determines its characteristics. We will use whichever model is most helpful to understand the concept being discussed.

THE ELECTROMAGNETIC SPECTRUM

Electromagnetic energy is all around us. X rays, gamma rays, radio waves, and light waves are forms of electromagnetic energy that we encounter every day. The only fundamental difference among them is the energy of the photons. The range of electromagnetic energy may be viewed as a spectrum, from lowest to highest energy. **Figure 1–2** shows some familiar forms of electromagnetic energy and their corresponding photon energies.

X-ray wavelengths are usually measured in nanometers (nm)—one of which is equal to one-millionth of a millimeter (mm). The useful range of medical radiography comprises wavelengths of approximately 0.01 to 0.05 nm. The wavelength of light in the center of the visible spectrum is about 550 nm, while the x rays used for radiography—those near the center of the medical x-ray spectrum—have a wavelength of approximately 0.05 nm or about 1/10,000 that of visible light. Remember that short wavelengths correspond to high energies.

Visible light is the form of electromagnetic radiation with which we are all most familiar. It is often helpful to use the analogy of visible light and x rays when answering questions from patients or staff about x-ray exposures. For example, it is commonly asked, "How long after the chest x-ray exposure do I have to wait until the x rays are gone from the room?" Or "Is the patient radioactive afterward?" X rays from a chest unit and visible light are both forms of electromagnetic radiation, electronically produced and controlled by a switch. You might respond with this analogy. Visible light disappears instantaneously from a room when the switch is shut off; x rays do the same. (People often get confused by the sound of the x-ray tube rotor, which may continue to coast long after the exposure is ended.) We also do not "glow" after the lights have been turned off in a room after being exposed to visible light. Similarly, patients who have been exposed during a diagnostic x-ray exam are not "radioactive" after their exam.

You might be wondering why we can "see" visible light, but cannot see x rays. Cells within the retina of the eye contain a special chemical called rhodopsin. When excited by electromagnetic energy in a certain range of energies, these cells send a signal to the brain, which we interpret as light. In fact, our perception of color is based on the fact that different colors of light have slightly different photon energies. Lower energy light photons are perceived as colors in the red-orange-yellow end of the visible light spectrum. Green-blue-violet colors represent higher energy light photons. The only reason why we cannot see x-radiation is because our eyes are not sensitive to photons with such high energies.

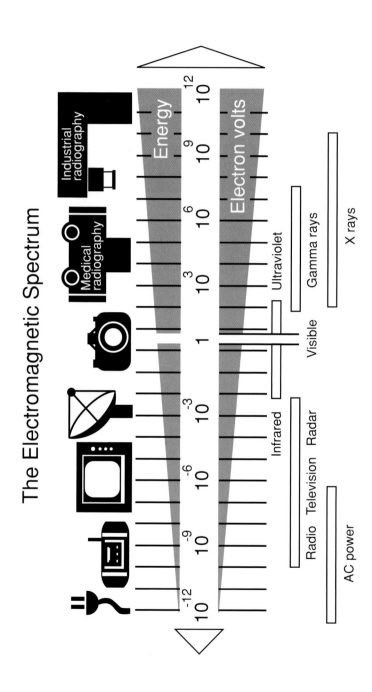

Figure 1–2 Electromagnetic Spectrum. The properties of electromagnetic radiation are determined by the energy of the photons. Photon energy (in electron volts) is shown increasing to the right.

FUNDAMENTAL PROPERTIES OF X RAYS

X rays have many properties in common with light. However, the unique properties of x rays are what make them invaluable in diagnostic imaging. Some of these are:

1. X rays are able to penetrate materials that absorb or reflect visible light.

2. When x rays are absorbed, they cause certain substances to *fluoresce*, that is, to emit radiation of lower energy (for example, visible and ultraviolet radiation).

3. Like light, x rays can produce an image on photosensitive film, such as photographic film or x-ray film, which can then be made visible by development.

4. Because of their high energy content, x rays can produce ions, that is, remove electrons from atoms to form positively charged ions and negative electrons. When formed and collected in a controlled manner, these ions may be used for measuring and controlling radiographic exposures.

When ions are formed in living tissue, there is a chance that they can produce biologic changes. When deliberately brought about by the use of high radiation doses, these biologic changes are used to treat tumors in radiation therapy. The substantially lower doses used in diagnostic imaging carry with them only a remote possibility of producing injury to humans. However, it is not a zero risk. Caution and care are the key approaches in the use of x-radiation.

These special properties are applied in medical and industrial radiography, radiation therapy, and research.

THE X-RAY SYSTEM

X rays used in medical radiography are electronically produced. **Figure 1–3** is a block diagram that depicts the major components of an x-ray system. The purpose of an x-ray system is to convert electrical energy into x-ray energy as specified by the user, and to direct the x rays toward the patient.

The x-ray **generator** converts the electrical power (provided by the local utility company) into high voltage power, which the x-ray tube requires to produce the x-ray beam. The generator converts the alternating current (AC) electrical power of 120, 208 and 220 volts into a waveform more suitable for the production of x rays. It also provides other forms of electrical power for the x-ray tube and other components of the x-ray system.

The **x-ray tube** converts the electrical energy provided by the generator into an x-ray beam. This is accomplished by imposing a high voltage between the negative cathode and the positive anode of the tube. Whenever electrons are produced at the negatively charged cathode and accelerated toward the anode, they strike the positively charged target area of the anode, and produce x rays **(Figure 1–4)**.

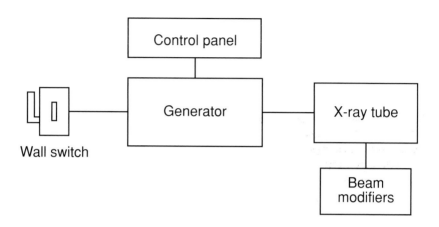

Figure 1–3 Simplified Block Diagram of a Typical X-ray Unit. An x-ray generator receives standard alternating current from a wall switch. A control panel is used to select the factors to make a radiograph. The generator provides the high-voltage waveform, according to the factors selected, that energizes the x-ray tube. Beam modifier attachments, including filtration, collimator, and cone are used to filter and shape the x-ray field.

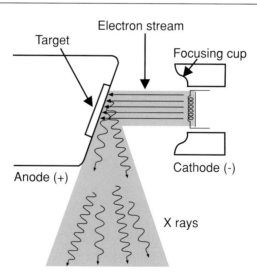

Figure 1–4 Emission of Electrons from the Heated Filament of the Cathode. When free electrons strike the stationary target of the anode, x-radiation is produced at the actual focal spot of the anode. Rays of different wavelengths and penetrating power are produced, shown schematically as lower energy (longer wavelength) and higher energy (shorter wavelength) x-ray photons.

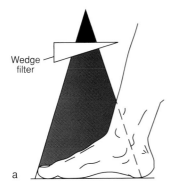

Wedge filter

a

Figure 1–5 Compensating X-ray Filtration **(a)** A compensatory filter (wedge) configured to the shape of the foot in the dorsoplantar position helps to produce an image with more uniform film blackening from the toes to the tarsal area. **(b)** Significant differences in thickness occur from the tip of the distal phalanges to the tarsal region of the foot. The measurements shown in this illustration are 2 cm at the toes and 8 cm in the tarsal region near the ankle. This represents a 1:4 ratio in tissue thickness.

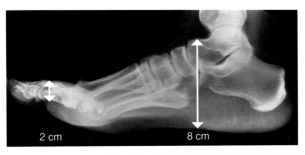

b   2 cm   8 cm

Most of the energy used in the production of x rays is converted to heat in the target. Less than 1% is typically converted into x-radiation.

The **control panel** is one of the two places where the x-ray machine operator can control the x-ray beam. Whether rudimentary or complex, the purpose of the control panel is to allow the operator to select predetermined settings of x-ray exposure and to initiate the exposure.

The second place where the x-ray machine operator can control the x-ray beam is at the **beam modifiers** (filter, collimator, cone or compensatory filter). These allow the operator to direct and limit the x-ray beam to the area of interest. Beam modifiers also provide the capability of altering the x-ray beam by introducing devices or accessories to shield radiosensitive areas of the patient, such as the gonads, breast, lens of the eye, and thyroid. **Compensatory filters** alter the x-ray beam to overcome the wide differences in film density arising from variations in anatomical thickness **(Figure 1–5)**.

The simplest example of a beam modifier is the **variable-aperture beam-limiting device**, commonly, but inaccurately referred to as a "collimator." This beam-limiting device consists of one or more lead shutters that restrict the beam to the size of the cassette or to the area of interest **(Figure 1–6)**. Positive Beam Limitation (PBL) devices automatically restrict the beam to the size of the cassette in use, but can be overridden if a smaller field size is indicated.

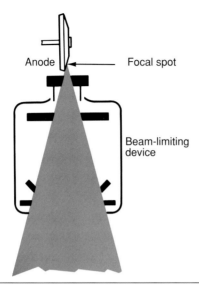

Anode — Focal spot

Beam-limiting device

Figure 1–6 Beam-Limiting Device. The x-ray beam from the x-ray tube passes through a beam-limiting device. The lead shutters within the collimator restrict the x-ray beam to a selected field size. After emerging from the device, the x-ray beam enters the part under examination.

GENERATORS

The purpose of the x-ray generator is to provide the power to the x-ray tube that is required to produce x rays, and to supply power to auxiliary components of the x-ray system. In the United States, utility companies supply 60 Hz AC power at certain selected voltages. A standard home or office electrical outlet provides approximately 120 volts AC, single-phase electrical energy. The term *alternating current* is used to describe a current waveform that is not constant, but changes its magnitude and direction of flow (polarity) in a sine-wave pattern **(Figure 1–7)**. The term AC is also used to describe a voltage with the same waveform. A standard AC outlet provides sufficient power for some x-ray applications, such as mobile radiography, dental and podiatry radiography, and some mammography.

Most x-ray generators are hard-wired directly into the electrical system, using 208 volts or higher, and most require a three-phase voltage supply.

To produce x rays, thousands of volts must be applied to an x-ray tube. The ideal type of voltage to be applied to the x-ray tube is a *constant voltage*. Since the utility supplies only AC power at a few hundred volts or less, the generator is designed to convert the supply power into a constant voltage, or at least nearly a constant voltage.

The two principal components in a generator are the transformer and the rectifier. A **transformer (Figure 1–8)** uses the principle of magnetic induction to change the magnitude of an AC voltage. An **auto-transformer** changes the voltage by a factor that is variable, usually controlled by a knob or an electric

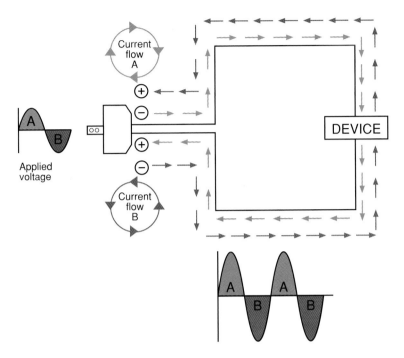

Figure 1–7 Alternating Current (AC) Electrical Power. Utilities supply 120 volts alternating current electrical power to energize electrical devices. Current flows through a complete circuit as negative electrons from the negative side of the power source are repelled by the negative voltage. These electrons are attracted towards the positive voltage of the power source. Alternating current changes in both magnitude and polarity (direction) 60 times per second. During the first half-cycle (gray, A) (1/120th second), the upper wire from the plug is negative with respect to the lower wire; current flows in a clockwise pattern. During the second half-cycle (red, B), the lower wire is negative, the upper wire positive, and current flows in a counterclockwise direction. This is an example of single-phase power.

motor. For example, if the operator selects a 100 volt setting from an auto-transformer energized from a 120 volt outlet, 100 volts are made available. A transformer is then used to step up (multiply) the voltage by a constant factor. If the 1000:1 step-up transformer shown in **Figure 1–8** were connected to the 100 volt output of the auto-transformer, 100,000 volts (or 100 kVp) would be produced. In this simple example, we have used two transformers to convert ordinary household line voltage into a voltage that can be applied to an x-ray tube to perform radiographic procedures, such as chest imaging.

The second principal component of an x-ray generator is a rectifier. A **rectifier** is a tube or semiconductor device that allows current to flow in one direction only (**Figure 1–9**). (Recall the alternating flow pattern of AC current shown in **Figure 1–7**.) In a way, an x-ray tube is a rectifier, since it allows current to flow only

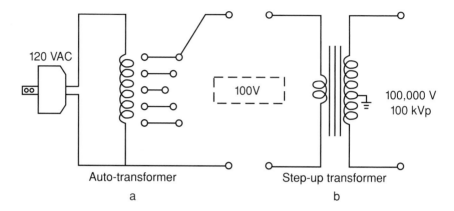

Figure 1–8 Auto-Transformer and Step-Up Transformer.   Different voltage levels can be tapped from an auto-transformer **(a)** to be used at the primary of the step-up transformer **(b)** to produce kilovoltage during the x-ray exposure. A step-up transformer is used to "step-up" voltage to kilovoltage. When 100 volts is applied to the primary of a step-up transformer with a 1000:1 ratio, 100,000 volts (100 kVp) results.

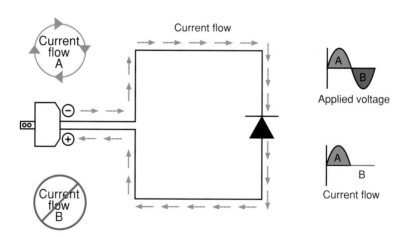

Figure 1–9 A Simple Rectification Circuit.   A rectifier permits current to flow in one direction only. In a simple rectification circuit, an AC power source energizes a rectifier. A single solid-state rectifier is shown with a negative voltage applied to the upper wire of the power supply (gray). Note that in the first half-cycle (A), the upper wire is negative and current flows clockwise. In the second half-cycle, the voltage polarity reverses (B), but the rectifier does not permit current to flow in the counterclockwise direction (red).

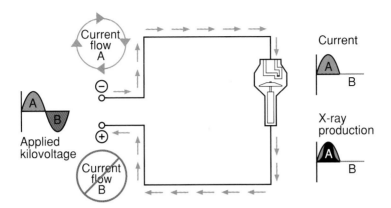

Figure 1–10 Self-Rectified X-ray Circuit. A self-rectified x-ray circuit is usually used for mobile, dental or podiatric x-ray units. AC voltage (60 Hz), supplied through a wall switch, has been stepped up to the kilovoltage range represented schematically by the alternating forward polarity (A) and reverse polarity (B) kilovoltage waveforms. In the first half-cycle (A), current flows from the negative side (gray) to the filament of the x-ray tube, across to the anode and back to the positive side of the power supply (red) and x rays are produced (solid wave). During the second half-cycle (B), the x-ray tube anode is negative with respect to the cathode; no current flows and no x rays are produced. This is also called half-wave rectification since only half of the voltage waveform is used to produce x-radiation.

when the cathode is negative and the anode is positive. In the first half-cycle, the cathode is negative with respect to the anode; this allows current to flow and x rays to be produced. During the second half-cycle, the cathode is positive and the anode is negative; therefore, no current flows and no x rays are produced. This is called a *self-rectified x-ray circuit* (**Figure 1–10**).

While this scenario demonstrates a simple (and inexpensive) method of producing x rays, it is clearly inefficient because half of the electrical power is not used. If the voltage applied to the x-ray tube were a constant voltage, with the cathode always negative and the anode always positive, the situation would be greatly improved. Specialized rectifier circuits are employed to bring about this improvement.

Figure 1–11 shows the next level of sophistication in x-ray generator circuits, the full-wave rectifier. In this circuit diagram, electrons can only flow in one direction through the rectifier (triangle symbol).

During the first half-cycle, electrons flow from the negative side of the voltage source (the upper terminal) through rectifier 4, through the x-ray tube (cathode-to-anode), through rectifier 2 and back to the lower (positive) terminal to complete the circuit. Rectifiers 1 and 3 do not allow current to flow through them during the first half-cycle.

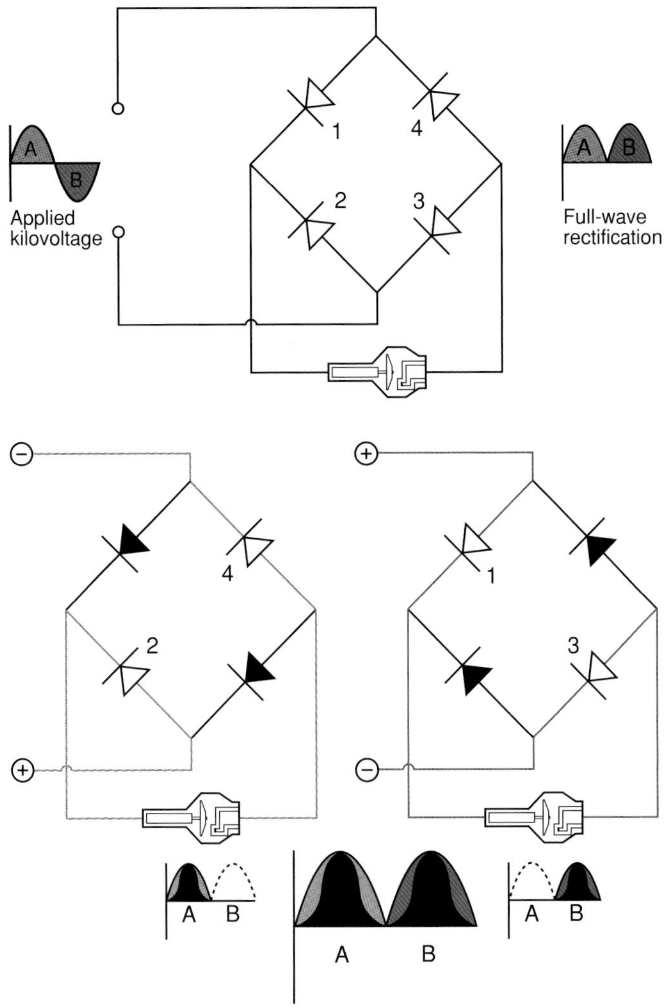

Figure 1–11 Full-Wave Rectification.   A full-wave rectification system is shown using four solid-state rectifiers (1–4). The AC applied kilovoltage waveform illustrates the forward polarity (A) and the reverse polarity (B) portion of the cycle. During the forward polarity portion of the cycle (gray), the current flows from negative to positive, through rectifier 4, to the x-ray tube from cathode to anode, and back through rectifier 2 to the opposite side of the transformer, and x rays are produced (solid). During the second half-cycle, the polarity reverses. Current always flows from negative to positive. The current flows through rectifier 3 (red), back to the tube from cathode to anode, and back through rectifier 1 (red) to the opposite side of the transformer. X rays are again produced. This is known as full-wave rectification because it utilizes full-voltage waveform to produce x rays. Efficiency of x-ray production increases as kilovoltage increases. This is shown in the solid areas of the waveforms (bottom).

During the second half-cycle, polarity is reversed. Electrons flow from the negative side of the voltage source (now the lower terminal) through rectifier 3, through the x-ray tube (cathode-to-anode), through rectifier 1 and back to the upper terminal to complete the circuit. Now, rectifiers 2 and 4 do not permit current to flow. This cycle is repeated 60 times per second (60 Hz).

Since current flows and x rays are produced during both half-cycles, the efficiency of the system has been substantially improved. This circuit produces a full-wave rectified waveform. While the full-wave circuit provides a substantial improvement in efficiency by using both halves of the power cycle, the resulting waveform is not at all close to the constant voltage that is optimum. The term *percent ripple* is used to quantify how close a voltage waveform is to constant. The percent ripple is defined as:

100 x (Maximum Voltage – Minimum Voltage)/Maximum Voltage.

The full-wave rectified circuit has 100% ripple. A constant voltage has 0% ripple (**Figure 1–12**).

The next improvement in x-ray generator waveforms uses three-phase AC power. In principle, three full-wave rectified circuits are connected to three-phase AC power, with the output of all circuits going to the x-ray tube. The result is a waveform with six-pulses per cycle (two for each half of the three phases) and about 13% ripple. A further enhancement of this design uses two sets of three-phase circuits, slightly out of phase with each other. The resulting three-phase, twelve-pulse waveform has only about 3% ripple, and is extremely close to the desired constant voltage (**Figure 1–12**).

High-Frequency Generators

Nearly all diagnostic x-ray generators made prior to 1980 used the 60 Hz frequency from the utility company to produce the kVp waveform applied to the x-ray tube. For single-phase equipment, the kVp waveform varies at the 60 Hz frequency. For three-phase equipment, the kVp waveform varies at a frequency that is a combination of three or more 60 Hz lines, separated from each other by slight delays. We say that they are "out-of phase" due to these delays. The result is a smoother kVp waveform (**Figure 1–12**).

The use of a higher frequency, generated by an electronic oscillator, has enabled manufacturers of x-ray equipment to build generators with the following attributes:

- much smaller than single-phase or three-phase generators,
- much less expensive to build, and
- tighter regulation of the kVp and tube current (mA) by the addition of closed-loop, electronic-feedback circuits.

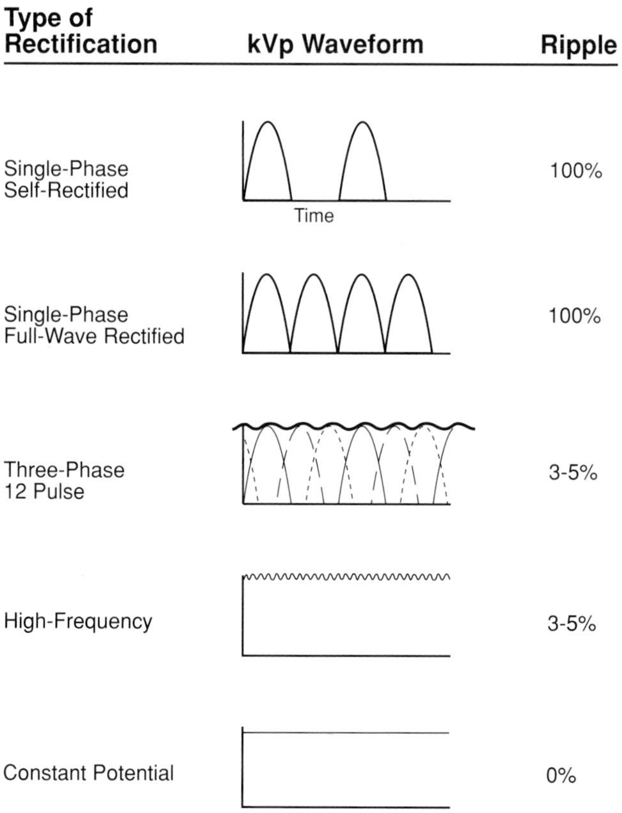

Type of Rectification	kVp Waveform	Ripple
Single-Phase Self-Rectified		100%
Single-Phase Full-Wave Rectified		100%
Three-Phase 12 Pulse		3-5%
High-Frequency		3-5%
Constant Potential		0%

Figure 1–12 Types of Waveforms and Ripple Factors. The percent ripple describes the maximum to minimum variation in the voltage waveform used to produce x rays, and is a function primarily of the type of rectification used in a generator. The waveforms and approximate corresponding percent ripple are shown for several different types of generators.

The frequencies used in high-frequency generators are in the range of 3,000 to as high as 100,000 Hz (100 kHz). The efficiency of transformers at these frequencies is much greater than at 60 Hz. An important result is that the high-tension transformer need not be as large as a conventional single- or three-phase transformer. Regulation of the kVp waveform and tube current in high-frequency generators is accomplished by the use of a *feedback circuit* (**Figure 1–13**). The kVp feedback circuit senses the difference between the tube kVp and the kVp set by the operator. The result is a voltage that is proportional to the difference. This voltage is input to a *voltage-controlled oscillator* (VCO). The VCO provides a correction to the original frequency used to generate the kVp and therefore can provide close regulation of the selected kVp.

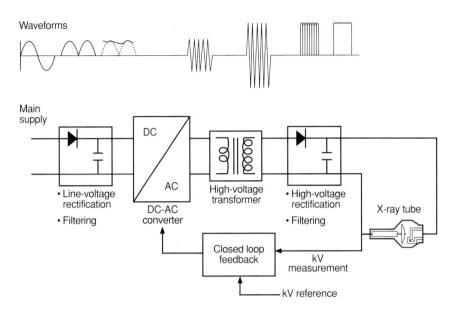

Figure 1–13 High-Frequency Generator. In a high-frequency generator, AC power is rectified and filtered, then passed through a DC/AC converter to produce a high-frequency AC waveform. The high-frequency waveform is stepped up by a high-voltage transformer. The high-voltage waveform is rectified and filtered, then applied to the x-ray tube. A closed-loop, electronic-feedback circuit is used for close regulation of kV. The upper portion of this schematic demonstrates the appropriate waveforms that occur during this process.

While there are some limitations to this design, high-frequency generators are generally smaller, less expensive, and better regulated than conventional designs. As a result, they are becoming increasingly popular in many diagnostic imaging applications.

Comparison of Generators

When comparing x-ray generators several compromises become obvious. Cost, size, efficiency, and power requirements must be weighed against the potential benefits of each type of generator.

Figure 1–12 summarizes waveform types and ripple factors. The ideal case is to have a constant voltage with 0% ripple. However, it is probably too simplistic to say that there is any one "ideal" type of generator; by design, each generator has its advantages and disadvantages. It is the responsibility of an informed user to select a generator with the best attributes (along with the most minimal disadvantages) for a particular application; cost is also an important consideration.

Single-Phase kVp	Three-Phase kVp
50	46
75	66
100	87
125	107
150	128

Figure 1–14 Generator Output Comparison. When making technique conversions from single-phase to three-phase generators, changes in kVp settings are usually required to obtain similar radiographic contrast and optical density.* Three-phase equipment requires lower kVp values than single-phase equipment to produce equivalent radiographic exposures.

*Optical density is discussed in detail in Chapter 5. Prior to establishing the definition of optical density, the intuitive term "film blackening" will be used.

The x-ray beam produced by a three-phase generator differs from that produced by a single-phase generator in the following ways.

1. The average x-ray *energy* produced by a three-phase generator is higher than for a single-phase generator for the same kVp setting. This means that if a desired x-ray exposure requires a 100 kVp setting from a single-phase generator, an equivalent x-ray exposure would be obtained by using 87 kVp on a three-phase generator (**Figure 1–14**). At a given kVp, the x-ray beam produced by a three-phase generator is more energetic and therefore more penetrating than one from a single-phase generator, other factors being equal.

2. The x-ray beam produced by a three-phase generator contains more *penetrating photons* than does the beam from a single-phase generator for the same kVp and mA setting. For example, using the same technique factors, a three-phase, six-pulse generator requires an exposure time approximately *two-thirds* that of a single-phase generator to produce the same blackness on film. For a three-phase, twelve-pulse generator, only about *one-half* the single-phase exposure time is needed.

3. The *heat load* on the anode is lower for a three-phase generator than for a single-phase generator to produce the same film blackening. This is of particular interest in angiography where, for a given kVp setting, approximately twice as many exposures can be made with a three-phase, twelve-pulse generator as with a single-phase generator, before the anode heat capacity of the tube is reached. Furthermore, with a twelve-pulse generator, it is possible to use shorter exposure times to reduce motion unsharpness in angiography.

THE X-RAY TUBE

When high-speed electrons collide with matter in any form, electromagnetic photons are produced. If the material is a metal with a high atomic number, and the electrons have sufficient energy (speed), x rays are produced.

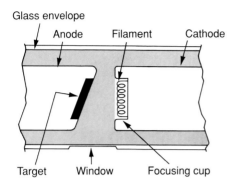

Glass envelope

Anode   Filament   Cathode

Target   Window   Focusing cup

Figure 1–15 Stationary-Anode X-ray Tube. The relationship of the filament in the focusing cup (cathode) to the target (anode) is shown.

The most efficient means of generating x rays is an x-ray tube. The simplest form of an x-ray tube uses a **stationary anode** housed in a sealed glass envelope from which air has been evacuated. Two important parts of the tube are the cathode and the anode **(Figure 1–15)**. In an x-ray tube, a "cloud" of electrons is produced at the filament wire and repelled by the negative charge of the cathode. The electron stream is shaped by the **focusing cup** and is attracted at high speed to the positively charged metal target area of the anode **(Figure 1–16)**. As the electrons interact with the atoms of the target, the electrons give up most of their energy in the form of heat. In medical radiography, only about 1% of their energy is emitted as x-radiation.

Cathode (−)

The cathode (negative electrode) contains a tungsten wire (filament) wound in the form of a coil about 1.5 mm in diameter and 10 to 15 mm long. The filament is mounted in a holder, called the focusing cup, about 2.5 cm [1 inch] or so away from the anode. Modern x-ray tubes contain two filaments, a small and a large, which are required to produce a small and a large focal spot (see line-focus principle in this chapter).

The filament is heated to a glow (incandescence) in the same way as a filament in an ordinary light bulb. It is not, however, heated to produce light, but to act as a source of electrons, which are emitted from the hot wire **(Figure 1–16)**. The length and diameter of the filament coil, the shape and size of the focusing cup, and their relative positions are factors that affect the shape and size of the spot where the electrons strike the anode. The temperature of the filament controls the quantity of electrons emitted from it. As the temperature is raised, more electrons are emitted; when kilovoltage is applied between the cathode and anode, the flow of electrical current through the x-ray tube (mA) begins.

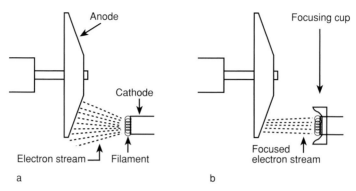

Figure 1–16 Electron Flow from Cathode to Anode. Most x-rays tubes have two filaments. These filaments are used to produce two different electron streams focused to a narrow rectangle on the anode (a single filament is shown here). A smaller filament produces an electron stream with a smaller cross-sectional area and therefore a smaller focal spot. **(a)** In this illustration, the electron stream is spread over a large area of the anode, due to the absence of a focusing cup. **(b)** When a (negatively charged) focusing cup is used, the electron stream is confined to a smaller area of the anode. The focusing cup keeps the electron stream from expanding due to the mutual electrostatic repulsion among the electrons.

Anode (+)

Anodes may be either stationary or rotating. A stationary anode (positive electrode) is usually formed from a block of copper. A plate of tungsten about 10 to 15 mm [about 1/2 inch] square and 3 mm thick is set in the anode face at the center of the tube. This is called the **target** and is generally made of tungsten because it has a high melting point (about 3400 °C), enabling it to withstand the extreme heat to which it is subjected. Tungsten also has a high atomic number (74) and is therefore a more efficient producer of x rays than materials of lower atomic numbers. The small area of the target that the electrons strike is called the **actual focal spot** or source and is the origin of x-radiation.

In specialized applications, targets of other materials such as molybdenum are used.

X-ray Production

When a very high electrical potential (kilovoltage) is applied across the x-ray tube—between the cathode and the anode—the free electrons are attracted to the anode in such a manner that they strike the focal spot with tremendous energy. Their path is illustrated in **Figure 1–16**. The higher the potential (voltage), the greater the energy (speed) of these electrons. High voltage results in x rays that are higher in energy and have greater penetrating power than that of x rays generated at lower voltages. Because x-ray tubes are more efficient at higher kilovoltages, x-ray output increases with increasing kVp.

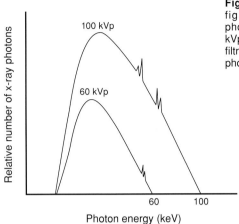

Figure 1–17 Energy Spectrum. This figure shows the spectra of x-ray photons produced at 100 kVp and 60 kVp, using a tungsten target and typical filtration. Note the tremendous range of photon energies within each beam.

Electrons that have the same energy when they reach the focal spot may produce x rays with different energies. This variation in x-ray energy, referred to as the x-ray spectrum, arises from differences in the ways individual electrons interact with the atoms of the target. The composition of the spectrum is determined by the target material, the kilovoltage and waveform applied to the tube, and the beam filtration. As higher kilovoltage is applied to the x-ray tube, the number of more energetic x-ray photons increases. The highest energy x rays are produced when all of the energy of the electron is converted into x-ray energy. All remaining x-ray photons in the beam have less energy. The applied kilovoltage also corresponds to the maximum energy photon produced. For example, 100 kVp applied across a tungsten-target tube produces a 100 kVp beam. Such a beam is composed of many photons of different energies (the highest of which has 100 kiloelectron volts [keV]), the distribution of which is characteristic of its tungsten-target spectrum **(Figure 1–17)**.

Most commonly, the kVp is selected for a given x-ray tube for a given patient examination. Sometimes, different desired spectra are selected by using x-ray tubes with different target materials.

Heat Production

The impact of the electrons generates heat as well as x rays. This heat must be removed from the anode as efficiently as possible. Otherwise, the metal anode would melt and the tube would be destroyed.

X-ray tubes are backed with a good heat-conducting metal to facilitate cooling by conduction and radiation. In addition, the tube is enclosed in a metal housing containing oil into which the heat of the anode is transferred.

The *actual focal spot* is the area of the target that is bombarded by the stream of electrons from the heated filament. The size of the filament coil and the shape and size of the focusing cup in which the coil is located are factors that affect the shape and size of the focal spot. The smaller the dimensions of the electron stream, the smaller the area of the target bombarded (actual focal spot) (**Figure 1–18**).

The size of the focal spot (source of x-radiation) has a very important effect upon the formation of the x-ray image. The smaller the focal spot, the sharper the image (other things being equal). However, a large focal spot can tolerate more heat than a small one. Therefore, methods for obtaining a focal spot that will provide good image detail and good heat dissipation must be found. Explained below are the line-focus principle and rotation of the anode during an exposure, which are the methods used to meet these needs.

Line-Focus Principle

The actual focal-spot size appears (and behaves) smaller when viewed from the position of the detector (film) because of the angle of the target to the electron stream. This effect is called the **line-focus principle**. As one would expect from the shapes of the focusing cup and filament (**Figure 1–16b**), the electron stream is focused in a narrow rectangle on the target. However, the target face is usually positioned at an angle of about 10° to 15° to the central ray of the primary beam (**Figure 1–18**). Consequently, when the rectangular focal spot is viewed from the position of the film, it appears more nearly a small square, which is known as the **projected** or **effective focal spot**. For this reason, the effective or projected area of the focal spot is only a fraction of its actual area on the target; and the smaller the target angle, the smaller the effective focal spot (other things being equal). This is illustrated in **Figure 1–18** where the effective focal-spot size for a 10° target angle is smaller than for a 15° target angle. Radiographic definition is improved, and the focal-track heat capacity of the anode is increased because the electron stream is spread over a greater area of the angled target. However, there is a practical limit to how small this angle can be. Use of too small an angle may cause an unacceptable reduction in x-ray output toward the anode side of the x-ray beam, thereby accentuating what is called the *heel effect*. (For an explanation of the heel effect, see Chapter 2.) As the anode angle is decreased, the field or area covered by the x-ray beam decreases in size.

Most tubes contain two separate filaments in a focusing cup, which provide two focal-spot sizes and the capacity to accommodate a variety of techniques and examinations (**Figure 1–18**).

In designating focal-spot size, manufacturers use a dimension known as the nominal focal-spot size. That is, a so-called 1.0 mm focal spot has a projected or *effective focal spot* that may differ from its nominal size by 50% or more,

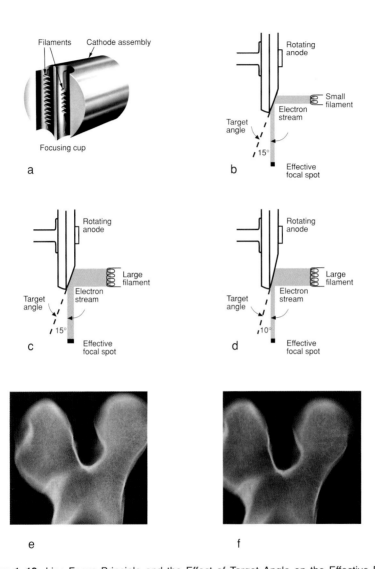

Figure 1–18 Line-Focus Principle and the Effect of Target Angle on the Effective Focal Spot. **(a)** A cathode assembly is shown with a small and large filament in a focusing cup. **(b)** An electron stream from the small filament results in a small effective focal spot. **(c)** A large electron beam from the large filament results in a large effective spot. **(d)** When a steep-angle target (10°) is used, the larger electron stream from the larger filament produces a smaller effective focal spot similar to that found in b. For the same effective focal spot, a steep-angle target distributes the heat from the electron stream over a larger area, and allows higher individual exposures than the conventional 15° targets. A 1 cm-thick transverse section of the distal femur of a cow is used to demonstrate the effect of small and large focal spots on bony trabeculation. **(e)** A small focal spot results in a high-resolution image with minimal image blur. **(f)** An image made with a large focal spot demonstrates increased image blur.

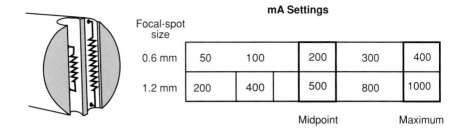

Focal-spot size	ma Settings				
0.6 mm	50	100	200	300	400
1.2 mm	200	400	500	800	1000
			Midpoint		Maximum

Figure 1–19 Focal-Spot Blooming. A 0.6 mm (small) and 1.2 mm (large) focal spot are indicated with typical milliampere settings. Note that the maximum setting of this small focal spot is 400 mA, 100% of the focal-spot rating. The larger focal spot can tolerate 1000 mA at maximum load. When the 400 mA setting is used on the small focal spot, the tube is operating at maximum output, therefore, focal-spot blooming may occur. When the same setting (400 mA) is used on the large focal spot, the x-ray tube is operating at below 50% of its maximum load, and focal-spot blooming is less of a concern. The 200 mA and 500 mA settings represent the midpoint output of the respective focal spots. Focal-spot blooming may occur when the maximum mA setting is used, particularly with a small focal spot at a lower kVp value.

according to tolerances permitted by the National Electrical Manufacturers' Association (NEMA).[1]

Focal-spot size can also be affected by exposure conditions. For instance, the focal spot tends to increase in size ("bloom") at higher mA settings, particularly at lower kVp settings. The selection of a small focal spot at maximum available mA may not provide the image sharpness expected with the small focal spot **(Figure 1–19)**.

There is increasing interest in tubes with very small focal spots (nominal diameters of about 0.1 mm) for use in magnification radiography, particularly mammography. When used with proper exposure factors, very small focal spots minimize geometric blurring, which is a limiting factor in magnification technique.

Rotating Anode

So far, a stationary-anode tube has been described. Because of the limitations of heat dissipation and focal-spot size associated with stationary anodes, their use in medical radiography is restricted mainly to low-output mobile, dental, and podiatric units. To increase the capacity of the anode to withstand heat, the rotating-anode tube was developed **(Figure 1–20)**. As the name implies, the disk-shaped anode (approximately 3 to 4 in. in diameter), composed of tungsten, molybdenum or sometimes graphite (upon which tungsten or a tungsten-rhenium alloy has been bonded), rotates on an axis through the center of the tube. The filament is positioned so that the electron stream can be attracted to the beveled area of the tungsten disk. The actual focal spot (the area of the target the electrons strike) remains in a fixed position while the anode disk rotates rapidly during

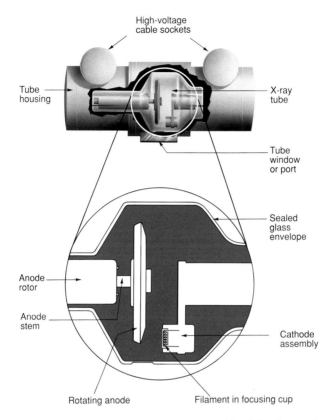

High-voltage
cable sockets

Tube
housing

X-ray
tube

Tube
window
or port

Sealed
glass
envelope

Anode
rotor

Anode
stem

Cathode
assembly

Rotating anode   Filament in focusing cup

Figure 1–20 Modern Rotating-Anode Tube. The relationship of the filament in a focusing cup (cathode) to the rotating anode is shown.

exposure (3,000 to 10,000 rpm), continually providing a cooler surface for the electron stream. In this way, the heat is distributed over the area of a broad ring or *focal track*. Consequently, for the same exposure conditions, the focal spot can be made significantly smaller than that in stationary-anode tubes.

The heat capacity of the anode and the intensity of the electron stream it can accommodate can be increased by making the diameter of the rotating disk larger. This allows the heat resulting from electron interactions to be spread out over a longer focal track and provides increased mass for heat absorption **(Figure 1–21)**.

The spindle (stem) on which the anode disk is mounted is usually made of molybdenum **(Figure 1–20)**. Molybdenum offers the advantages of strength, high melting point and low thermal conductivity, which reduces heat flow from the anode to the rotor and bearings. Current technology permits anodes to be operated continuously at extremely high temperatures. At these temperatures, most of the heat is transferred by radiation (instead of conduction) to the oil

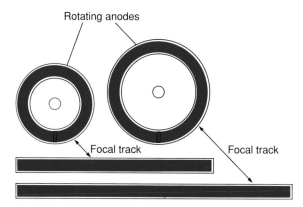

Figure 1–21 The Effect of the Anode Diameter on Focal Track Length. Face view of two rotating anodes of different diameters. A larger diameter anode results in a longer focal track, which can tolerate higher individual exposures as well as increased heat unit capacity.

surrounding the tube and tube housing. For tubes designed for heavy-duty usage, such as for angiography and computed tomography, the oil from the tube housing is often circulated through a heat exchanger.

X-ray tubes should always be operated within their rated capacities and only after the manufacturer's recommended warm-up procedure. Manufacturers furnish charts with all x-ray tubes to indicate the limits of safe operation. Single-exposure tube rating charts indicate the maximum kilovoltage, milliamperage, and time that can be safely used for a single exposure. Tube cooling charts are also available, which indicate how rapidly exposures may be repeated (anode thermal characteristics). Tube housing cooling characteristics are also available from the manufacturer.

TECHNIQUE FACTOR SELECTIONS

In the most simple systems, the operator selects the characteristics of the x-ray exposure (technique factors) by selecting the *output* of the generator, that is, the duration of exposure (seconds or fractions of a second), kilovoltage (kVp), and milliamperage (mA). Other generators combine the exposure time and mA into a single quantity known as mAs (mAs = mA x s, where *s* is in seconds or fractions of a second).

Kilovoltage

The peak kilovoltage (kVp) is the maximum voltage applied to the x-ray tube. *Increasing the kVp increases the energy (speed) of the electrons as they are accelerated across the x-ray tube. Therefore, the kVp setting controls the penetrating power of the x rays.* Higher kVp settings produce more penetrating x rays and radiographs with lower subject contrast, which will be explained in more detail later.

Milliamperage

Milliamperage (mA) is a measure of the number of electrons flowing per second across the x-ray tube during an exposure. One milliampere equals 1/1,000 ampere. The number of free electrons is controlled by the temperature (the degree of incandescence) of the cathode filament. This control is accomplished by adjusting the filament current through its own low-voltage electric circuit. Setting the x-ray machine for a specific mA actually means adjusting the filament temperature. The hotter the filament, the more electrons available to form the electron stream, that is, the tube current (mA). For example, if the number of electrons per second doubles, the current (mA) doubles and the x-ray output doubles.

When the mA is multiplied by the time of exposure (seconds or fractions of a second), the result is mAs (milliampere-seconds). The number of x-ray photons produced at a particular kilovoltage depends upon the milliampere-seconds (mAs). *For a given kVp setting, the amount of x-radiation produced increases linearly with mAs.*

Some generators offer the capability of automatic exposure control (AEC), in which the operator selects the kVp and an electronic circuit automatically terminates the exposure when the film has received a preset amount of radiation. Because patients vary in their absorption of x rays (primarily due to thickness and density), this provides a convenient means of avoiding radiographs that are under- or overexposed (too light or too dark). More sophisticated systems offer the capability to preprogram the technique factors for a given exam, such as those used for an "average" chest radiograph or a "dense" breast in mammography.

RADIATION SAFETY

Radiation can be hazardous to humans if not used carefully. This situation is similar in many ways to electricity; if standard safety procedures are ignored, serious injury can result from many plug-in appliances. However, by knowing and following accepted safety procedures, most of us use electricity without injury every day of our lives.

While it is beyond the scope of this book, it is worth emphasizing that proper safety procedures must always be followed when using x-radiation to prevent injury to patients and staff. Users must know and follow the radiation safety procedures (both institutional and statutory) that apply to their environment.

SUMMARY

X rays are a form of electromagnetic radiation with sufficiently high energy to penetrate matter. The x-ray system consists of a control panel, generator, x-ray tube, and beam modifying devices. Beam modifying devices allow the operator to shape and alter the x-ray beam to meet the varied requirements of medical radiography. The control panel allows the operator to select the desired technique factors for an x-ray exposure.

The simplest type of x-ray generator uses a self-rectified x-ray circuit with a high-voltage transformer to provide the kilovoltage needed by the x-ray tube for x-ray production. More sophisticated types of generators deliver a kVp waveform with reduced ripple for greater x-ray production efficiency.

X rays are produced in an x-ray tube when electrons from the filament are accelerated from the cathode to the target (anode). In the target, high energy electrons interact with high atomic number elements to produce x rays.

Appropriate radiation safety procedures must be established and followed to protect the operator and the patient from unnecessary x-ray exposure and the risk of associated health effects.

Chapter 2
The X-ray Beam and Image Formation

X rays, like visible light, radiate from their source in straight lines in all directions until they are stopped by an absorber or are scattered (**Figure 2–1**). For this reason, the x-ray tube is enclosed in a lead-lined metal housing that stops most of the x-radiation. Only a small cone of useful x-rays leaves the tube through a window or port in the housing. These useful rays are termed the **primary beam**, the geometric center of which is called the **central ray**.

In most medical x-ray machines, kilovoltage can be varied over a fairly wide range—usually from 40 kVp to 125 kVp or more. When lower kilovoltages are used, the x rays have lower energies and are more easily absorbed by structures within the patient. These are sometimes referred to as "soft" x rays. Radiation produced at higher kVp has greater energy. This relatively more penetrating radiation is sometimes called "hard" radiation. X-ray beams used in medical radiography are heterogeneous or polyenergetic, in that they consist of radiation of different energies and penetrating powers.

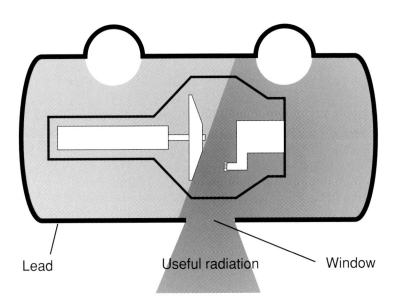

Lead   Useful radiation   Window

Figure 2-1 Radiation of X rays from X-ray Tube Target. X rays radiate from the source (target) of the x-ray tube in all directions. A protective, lead-lined metal housing encloses the x-ray tube, allowing the useful portion of the x-ray beam to exit from the tube window.

X-RAY ABSORPTION

One of the useful properties of x rays is their ability to penetrate matter. However, if every x-ray photon that entered an object were to penetrate it, x-ray imaging would be impossible as we know it. The resulting radiograph would be completely and uniformly black, and would convey no information about the structure of the object under study. Some x-ray photons are absorbed by structures within the patient, while others penetrate the patient and reach the image receptor to produce a useful medical radiographic image.

Consider radiography of the test object in **Figure 2–2**. Region A consists of a very thin sheet of plastic wrap, region B, a 1 cm block of aluminum, and region C, a 10 cm block of lead that absorbs every x-ray photon.

Assume that the entire test object is exposed to a uniform beam of x rays with an **x-ray fluence*** of 100 x-ray photons per square centimeter. Region A is so thin that all of the x rays that reach the plastic wrap are transmitted and reach the image receptor. One would say that this section of the film is exposed to 100 photons/cm². Another way of describing this is to say that the film is exposed to an x-ray fluence of 100 photons/cm².

Region B absorbs some (but not all) of the x rays that reach the aluminum block. If region B had a 50% absorption of the x rays, the x-ray fluence reaching the film would be 50 photons/cm².

The block of lead (object C) absorbs 100% of the x rays to which it is exposed and therefore the film is exposed to a fluence of 0 photons/cm². **Figure 2–3** repeats the same test object and x-ray beam exposure as **Figure 2–2** with the exception of a penny added to the top of both the aluminum and lead blocks.

These simplified examples provide the following useful insights into radiographic imaging.

1. The area of the film under object A in both **Figure 2–2 and 2–3** will be completely black after processing because all of the x rays reach the film. (Every time an x-ray photon exposes the film, some film blackening occurs.)

2. The area of the film under object C in **Figure 2–2** will be completely white because no x rays were able to penetrate the lead and expose the film.

3. The area of the film under object B in **Figure 2–2** will be some intermediate shade of gray. Shades of gray are produced when there are sufficient x-ray photons to partially expose the film, but not enough to make it completely black.

4. The radiograph in **Figure 2–3** provides very little information about the structure of object C. For example, whether some parts of object C were slightly thicker than others. Or if someone placed a penny on top of the object, the radiograph provides no information about the penny. Since not a single photon reached the film, there is really not much information in this section of the radiograph.

---

*Fluence may be defined as the number of photons per unit area. Actual x-ray photon fluences would be many millions of photons/cm², but lower numbers are used for simplicity.

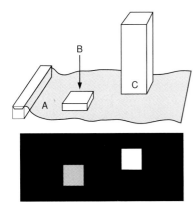

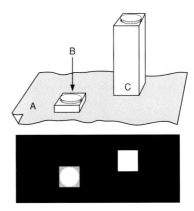

Figure 2–2 The Effect of Various Materials on the Absorption of X rays. Test objects include a plastic wrap (**A**), a 1 cm block of aluminum (**B**), and a 10 cm block of lead (**C**). The plastic wrap is so thin that even the smallest amount of x-radiation used in an exposure passes through unattenuated to reach the image receptor. The aluminum block absorbs some but not all of the x-radiation reaching it, and is imaged as a gray pattern adjacent to the blackened area of the radiograph. Because of the high atomic number of lead (82) and its 10 cm height, 100% of the x-ray beam is absorbed. The lead is seen as a white square against a black background.

Figure 2–3 An Example of the Effect of X-ray Absorption on the Imaging of Structures within Objects. This illustration duplicates the setup in **Figure 2–2** with the exception of the position of a penny on top of the aluminum block (**B**), and a second penny on top of the lead block (**C**). Note that some of the x-ray photons reach the detector in object B outlining the shape of the penny. X-ray photons penetrate the penny but not the block of lead (**C**), therefore, the outline of this penny is not seen.

5. The radiograph in **Figure 2–3** does, however, provide useful information about the structure of object B. If a penny had been left on top of this object, the added thickness of copper would have absorbed some additional photons, which would otherwise have reached the film. The fluence beneath the penny would be somewhat lower (perhaps 40 photons/cm^2) than the other areas of the aluminum block. As a result, the radiograph would contain a light circle, demonstrating the presence of the penny.

6. In order to produce a useful radiograph, some x rays must reach the film to produce film blackening. Nearby areas of the film exposed to a lower fluence have a lighter shade of gray, while areas exposed to a greater fluence appear darker. X-ray photons that do penetrate the object form the **aerial image**, also sometimes known as the **image in space**. This refers to the x-ray beam that exits the object of interest but has not yet reached the image receptor (film). The x-ray beam used to expose the test object has a constant photon fluence across the length and width of the x-ray beam; whereas the aerial image has a non-uniform fluence due to absorption differences within the object.

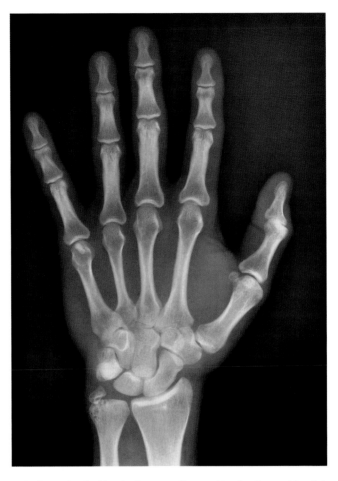

Figure 2–4 Radiograph of a Hand. A screen-film combination is capable of demonstrating many shades of gray, which provides information about structures under study. A radiograph of a hand demonstrates excellent soft tissue visualization, as well as bony trabeculation. The "whitest white" in the image represents the cortex of the bone, while the exposed areas around the hand represent the maximum blackening potential of the screen-film detector.

7. Radiographic film is capable of showing many shades of gray, thereby providing much information about the structure of objects under study. A useful radiograph takes advantage of many subtle shades of gray; it is neither too light, nor too dark (**Figure 2–4**).

8. In reality, absorption of x-radiation is not an "all-or-nothing" phenomenon as it is explained in **Figures 2–2 and 2–3**. X-ray absorption is a random process, like winning a lottery. Buying a single ticket does not guarantee that you will win, but the more tickets you buy, the greater the probability that you will win

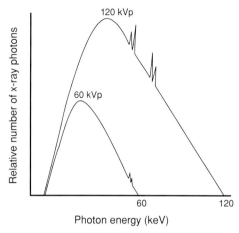

Figure 2–5 Energy Spectrum. The spectra of x-ray photons produced at 120 kVp and 60 kVp using a tungsten target and typical filtration are shown.

(even though that chance may be slim). When an x-ray photon is incident upon an object, there is a certain probability that it will be absorbed. When we say that an object is "more absorbing" than another, we mean that there is a higher probability of x-ray absorption.

The simplified examples in **Figure 2–2 and 2–3** ignore the effect of scattered radiation and several other complicating factors, which will be examined later in more detail.

FACTORS AFFECTING X-RAY ABSORPTION

X-ray absorption is a function of the spectrum of the x-ray beam and the characteristics of the absorbing material. The energy spectrum and absorbing material characteristics are determined by the following factors.

The Spectrum of an X-ray Beam

An x-ray beam is polyenergetic because it consists of a range of energies with different relative numbers of photons at each energy. The maximum photon energy present equals the **peak kilovoltage** (kVp) applied across the tube, although almost no photons have this ideal maximum energy. The term **spectrum** is used to describe *the relative number of x-ray photons produced by the target at a given energy, for a given type of x-ray tube.* A spectrum is often represented by the shape of a curve as seen in **Figure 2–5**. Here you see the x-ray spectra from a 60 kVp and a 120 kVp tungsten-target beam. Notice the tremendous range of photon energies within each beam. Generally speaking, higher energy x rays are more penetrating and therefore less easily absorbed (have a lower probability of

Filtration Comparison			
Tube Type	Target	Total Filtration	
		Inherent +	Added
Conventional	Tungsten rhenium	Glass window	Aluminum
Mammography	Molybdenum	Beryllium window	Molybdenum

Figure 2–6 Filtration Comparison. The target and filtration associated with conventional and mammographic tubes are compared.

absorption) than lower energy x rays. The spectrum of an x-ray beam is affected by kilovoltage, voltage waveform, target material, and beam filtration.

Kilovoltage

Raising the kVp changes the spectrum by increasing the maximum energy of x rays in the spectrum, producing an x-ray beam with more higher energy photons as well as more photons of all energies. Remember that higher energy photons in the spectrum produce an x-ray beam with greater penetration and less absorption in a given material. Therefore, increasing kVp decreases x-ray absorption.

Voltage Waveform

For a given setting, the average kilovoltage applied to the x-ray tube by a three-phase generator is higher than for a single-phase generator because of waveform differences. Therefore, changing from a single-phase to a three-phase generator has an effect on the energy spectrum of the x-ray beam that is somewhat similar to increasing the kVp. As with increased kVp, this effect changes the x-ray spectrum by increasing the proportion of higher energy photons in the beam and therefore it also decreases x-ray absorption.

Target Material

The spectrum or energy distribution of the x-ray beam is affected by the material from which the target is made. In most medical applications, the target of the x-ray tube is composed of tungsten or a tungsten-rhenium alloy. For some special applications, for instance mammography, other materials such as molybdenum are used to provide specific advantages in subject contrast or dose reduction. The characteristic shape of the x-ray spectrum is determined by the combination of target and filtration materials. The target material determines the distribution of x-ray photon energies *produced*; the filtration material determines the distribution of photon energies (shape of the spectrum) that *penetrate* the filter and ultimately comprise the x-ray beam incident on the patient.

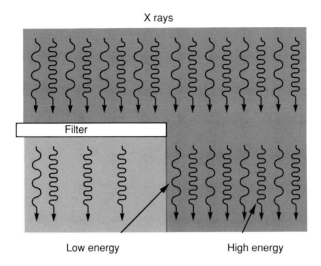

Figure 2–7 The Effect of Filtration on the X-ray Beam. Note the different energies in the x-ray beam prior to reaching the filter, illustrated as different wavelengths. A filter removes more low-energy radiation (longer wavelengths) than it does high-energy radiation.

Filtration

Filtration is the preferential removal of lower energy photons from the x-ray beam by an absorber (filter). Filtration by such items as the glass wall of the x-ray tube and the insulating oil surrounding the tube are referred to as **inherent filtration**. A filter consisting of a sheet of metal inserted into the x-ray beam (usually aluminum in general medical radiography) is called **added filtration**. The **total filtration** in the beam is the sum of the inherent plus added filtration **(Figure 2–6)**.

The x-ray beam is composed of a spectrum of photons with different energies and penetrating powers. When a filter is introduced into the beam, it alters that spectrum. An aluminum filter added to a tungsten-target x-ray tube removes more of the lower energy, less-penetrating photons than it does of the higher energy photons **(Figure 2–7)**. This increases the overall penetrating power of the beam, as determined by the percentage of photons that reach the image receptor, without changing kVp.

To help in understanding the concept of beam filtration, consider this analogy of an advanced calculus class with 100 students initially enrolled. At the end of the semester, 60 students passed the course. Therefore, the percentage of students passing the course was 60/100 or 60%. Unfortunately, 10 of the students enrolled had never had any prior math courses, and would most likely fail the course. If the students had been screened for the course by requiring a prerequisite basic calculus course, those 10 students would never have been admitted to the

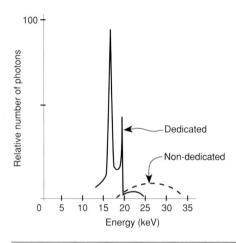

Figure 2–8 Typical X-ray Emission Spectra for Two Mammography Units. Spectra for dedicated and non-dedicated x-ray units are shown, normalized to unit area. The dedicated unit was used with a molybdenum target, 0.03 mm molybdenum filter, and 25 kVp setting. The non-dedicated unit was used with a tungsten-target tube, aluminum filtration, and 35 kVp setting.[3]

advanced course. If this screening process had been used, the same 60 students would have passed the course—this time out of only 90 enrolled students. This process of screening increased the passing percentage to 60/90 or 66%, and removed from the outset those students who would most likely never have passed the course.

This screening process is analogous to the "hardening" of an x-ray beam by the insertion of filters. Hardening an x-ray spectrum preferentially removes lower energy photons that would never reach the film to contribute to the image. Filtration increases the proportion of high-energy, more penetrating photons in the beam by filtering out lower energy photons.

Even at high-kilovoltage settings, the beam always contains some x rays of low energy (penetrating power). The probability is low that these low-energy x rays will pass through the patient's body and form a useful image. Most of this low-energy, *non-image forming radiation* will merely add to the dose absorbed by the patient. Therefore, it is desirable and, in fact, mandated by the Food and Drug Administration (FDA) that certain minimum amounts of filtration be placed in the beam.[2] This filtration must be added to remove the low-energy x rays that add to the patient's skin dose, but do not contribute to the image.

Filtration may be specified in terms of **aluminum equivalent** (the thickness of aluminum required to produce the same filtering action) or in terms of **half-value layer** *(HVL)*, that is, the thickness of material required to reduce beam fluence to one-half of its original value. Federal and state regulatory agencies and equipment manufacturers can supply further information about filtration requirements.

It is worth restating that the shape of the energy spectrum of an x-ray beam is a function of both the target and filtration materials. In mammography, for

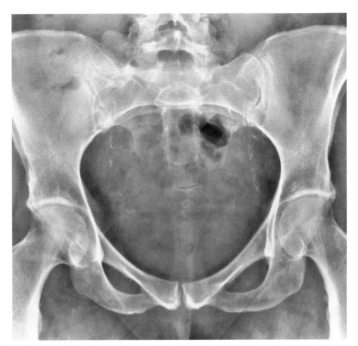

Figure 2–9 Radiograph of the Pelvis. An evenly exposed radiograph of a pelvis is possible since the pelvic structures are relatively uniform in thickness (absorption).

example, the selection of target and filter is based on factors other than simply increasing the penetrating power of the beam by removing lower energy photons. As the technical aspects of mammographic imaging became better understood, it became clear that selection of a molybdenum target with a molybdenum filter produced an x-ray beam with a spectrum particularly well-suited for mammography **(Figure 2–8).** More recently, it has been suggested that still other target-filter combinations may improve mammographic imaging under certain conditions.

Specialized target-filter combinations have not been limited to mammography, as they have been suggested to be of value in certain general imaging applications. Optimizing target-filter combinations is an area of ongoing research. Such combinations may continue to evolve in the years ahead. However, a good understanding of these concepts and their effect on the energy spectrum will enable the reader to evaluate proposed new technologies as they become available.

A relatively uniform x-ray beam seems well-suited to producing good radiographs of many structures, such as in the pelvis **(Figure 2–9).** In the previous example of **Figure 2–2**, a three-section test object was radiographed using an idealized x-ray beam in which the photon fluence was uniform across the length and width of the x-ray beam.

Another form of filtration uses non-metallic **compensators** to alter primarily the photon fluence of the beam. It is difficult to produce a quality radiograph of the foot because the foot is much thinner at the toes than at the ankle. Use of a uniform x-ray beam will result in a radiograph with overexposed toes and an underexposed ankle. In this case, a wedge-shaped aluminum or lead-loaded acrylic compensating filter is placed between the x-ray tube and the patient **(Figure 1-5)**. The thicker end of the compensatory filter absorbs or attenuates more x-radiation than the thinner end, producing an x-ray beam with a higher photon fluence at the thinner end of the filter. Judicious positioning of the compensating filter with respect to the foot yields a radiograph with more even density across the entire image.

Absorbing Material Characteristics

Thickness of the Absorber

The relationship between x-ray absorption and thickness is intuitively obvious—a thick piece of any material absorbs more x-radiation than a thin piece of the same material. For example, 15 cm of water will absorb more x rays than 3 cm of water.

Density of the Absorber

For materials that differ in density (mass per unit volume), for example, g/cm^3, higher density materials absorb more x-radiation than those of lower density, other things being equal. For example, 3 cm of water will absorb more x rays than 3 cm of steam because steam weighs less (has less mass) per cubic centimeter than water.

Atomic Number of the Absorber

The atomic number of the material of which the object is composed affects its x-ray absorption characteristics. In general, the lower the atomic number of a material, the less it absorbs x-radiation. For example, the atomic number of aluminum is 13; lead is 82. Therefore, a sheet of aluminum absorbs a smaller amount of x rays than does a thinner sheet of lead of the same area and weight. This is why lead is used in the tube housing and as a lining for the walls of x-ray rooms, as well as in protective gloves and aprons.

Contrast Media

In order to enhance absorption differences between body structures and the regions surrounding them, contrast media are sometimes introduced into these

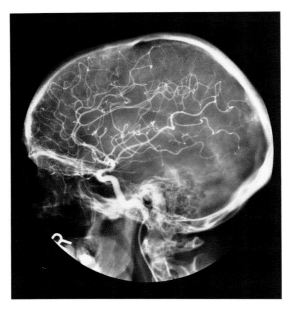

Figure 2–10 The Effect of Contrast Media on X-ray Absorption in a Cerebral Arteriogram. The arteries of the brain in this cerebral arteriogram are seen because they contain an iodinated compound (contrast media) that absorbs more x-radiation than the surrounding tissues of the brain.

structures. **Contrast media** are substances that differ in density and atomic number from the tissues surrounding the region into which they are introduced.

Some common substances used as contrast media are: aqueous suspensions of barium sulfate, liquid organic compounds containing iodine, and gases, such as air.

Barium sulfate and air are generally used to outline the gastrointestinal tract. Substances that absorb more x-radiation than their surroundings, such as barium sulfate, are said to be *radiopaque*. Substances that are less absorbing than surrounding tissue, such as air, are said to be *radiolucent*.

Iodinated contrast media has many uses, including radiography of the vascular and urinary systems, and the spinal canal. **Figure 2–10** shows a cerebral arteriogram in which the blood vessels containing an iodinated contrast medium are easily differentiated from surrounding structures because of the high absorption of x rays by iodine.

DIFFERENTIAL ABSORPTION IN THE HUMAN BODY

The human body is a complex subject for imaging, composed of not only different thicknesses but also different materials that absorb x rays in varying degrees. The essence of medical radiographic imaging is to expose a segment of the body to a relatively uniform fluence of x-radiation, which will be altered by structures within the patient. The resulting aerial image will contain all of the imaging information. But since our eyes are not sensitive to x rays, we must use an **image receptor**, such as a screen-film combination, to convert this aerial image into a visible light image that we can evaluate.

Radiographs of high quality can be produced when selected technical factors (kVp, mAs, target-filter combination, compensators, screen-film combination) take advantage of the differential absorption of x rays in the body.

Bone contains elements of higher atomic number than soft tissue. The density of bone is also somewhat higher than that of soft tissue. Therefore, bone absorbs more x rays than soft tissue. Furthermore, diseased structures often absorb x rays differently than do their healthy counterparts. The age of the patient can also have a bearing on absorption. In the elderly, bones may have less calcium content and therefore less x-ray absorption than bones of younger people.

The difference in absorption of bone and soft tissue is affected by the spectrum of the x-ray beam used. As the x-ray beam emerges from the body, the photon fluence of the entrance x-ray beam has been altered by the absorption effect of the body parts in the beam. Therefore, the aerial image is a pattern of differing photon fluences caused by interactions within the body.

Consider, for example, the x-ray fluences emerging from a body part consisting of bone surrounded by soft tissue, shown schematically as a cross section in **Figure 2–11**. The bone absorbs more x-radiation than the surrounding soft tissue because of its higher atomic number and density. Accordingly, the photon fluence under the bone is *less* than that under the soft tissue.

Subject Contrast

The ratio of the x-ray photon fluence emerging from one part of an object to the fluence emerging from a more absorbing adjacent part is called **subject contrast** (**Figure 2–12**). If the x-ray fluence under the soft tissue is 300 photons/cm² and the x-ray fluence in the area under the bone is 100 photons/cm², the photon fluence ratio is 3:1, in which case, the subject contrast would be 3.

Subject contrast depends upon the nature of the subject (thickness and composition) and the x-ray spectrum (kilovoltage, voltage waveform, filtration, and target material)—in other words, upon those factors that affect x-ray absorption—and upon the amount and distribution of scattered radiation (see Chapter 3). However, *subject contrast is independent of exposure time, milli-amperage, the characteristics and processing of the film and, for all practical purposes, distance.*

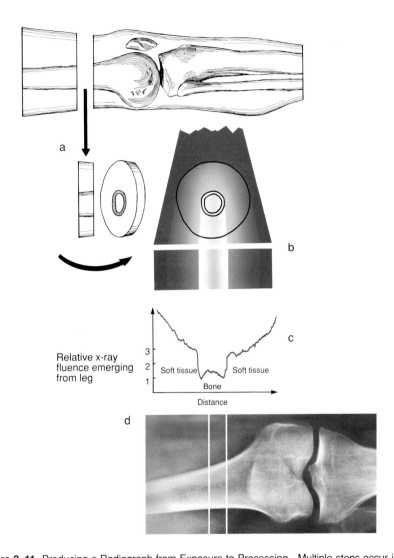

Relative x-ray
fluence emerging
from leg

Figure 2–11 Producing a Radiograph from Exposure to Processing. Multiple steps occur in the production of a radiograph beginning with exposure of the part under study. **(a)** A transverse section of the distal femur is shown rotated to illustrate the absorption effects of the tissues of the lower thigh. **(b)** The structures within the thigh cause a variation in the fluence of the incident x-ray beam to produce the aerial image, which is recorded on radiographic film as a latent image. As the x-ray beam passes through the leg, the fluence under the bone is lower than that under the soft tissue because bone absorbs more x-radiation than the surrounding soft tissue. **(c)** A graph is used to display the fluence variations across the x-ray beam emerging from the thigh. The fluence emerging from the soft tissue is three times greater than that from the bone. Therefore, the subject contrast between these structures is 3. **(d)** The transverse section is displayed in the AP radiograph.

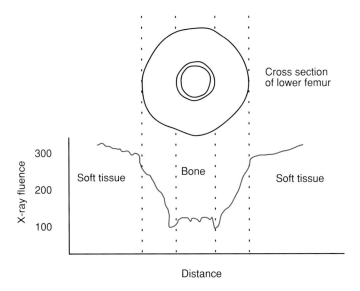

Figure 2–12 Representation of the Absorption Characteristics of a Body Part. Variations in x-ray absorption arising from bone and soft tissue are shown. Subject contrast may be determined from the arbitrary scale of x-ray fluence. A subject contrast of approximately 3:1 between soft tissue and bone is shown in the example.

Exposure Factors Affecting the Aerial Image

Some x-ray exposure factors affecting the aerial image (that is, the pattern of x-ray photon fluence emerging from the body incident on the image receptor) are: mAs, x-ray energy spectrum, and distance.

mAs

Increasing the mAs increases the overall fluence of the x rays produced. Therefore, as the mAs is increased, the x-radiation fluence arising from the focal spot increases. All the fluences in the pattern emerging from the body increase similarly, that is, the various x-ray fluences continue to bear the same relation to each other. For instance, in **Figure 2–12**, consider that initially 300 photons/cm^2 (fluence) are measured under the soft tissue alone and 100 photons/cm^2 are measured under the bone. Now consider that the mAs flowing through the x-ray tube is doubled, resulting in a doubling of x-ray output. Doubling the mAs also doubles the fluences emerging from the soft tissue and bone to 600 and 200, respectively. As a result, the ratio of 3:1 in subject contrast remains unchanged. In other words, the fluence under the soft tissue alone will always be three times that under the bone, whether the mAs is increased or decreased—other factors remaining unchanged. What has changed is the *total number of x-ray photons* used to expose the image receptor. Doubling the

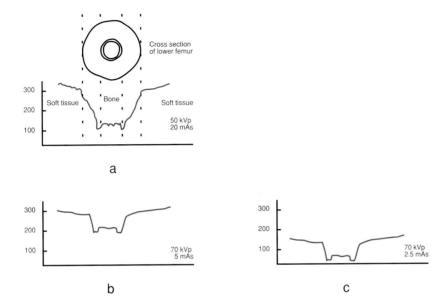

Figure 2–13 The Effect of Kilovoltage and Milliamperage on the Aerial Image. Graphs are used to illustrate the variation in x-ray fluence with position across the aerial image of the lower femur resulting from changes in kVp and mAs. Comparing the fluence distribution for a 50 kVp beam **(a)** with that of a 70 kVp beam **(b)** shows that as kVp is increased, fluence and penetrating power increase and subject contrast decreases from 3:1 to 3:2 in this hypothetical example. Comparison of the patterns resulting from reducing the mAs from 5 mAs **(b)** to 2.5 mAs **(c)** shows that the x-ray fluence has been halved, but that corresponding fluences bear the same relation to each other—300/200 (3:2) and 150/100 (3:2). That is, subject contrast is not changed by altering mAs for both b and c.

---

mAs produces twice as many total photons, which have a greater film blackening effect than the lower mAs. Therefore, *more mAs means darker radiographs, but subject contrast remains the same.*

Spectrum: kVp, Voltage Waveform, and Target-Filtration Combination

The spectrum of an x-ray beam may be altered by changing kVp, voltage waveform, and target-filter combination. Such changes also have an effect on subject contrast and overall film blackening.

When the x-ray spectrum is hardened (filtered) or the kVp is increased, the beam consists of more penetrating, higher energy x rays. The bone surrounded by soft tissue shown schematically in **Figure 2–12** is used again in **Figure 2–13** to illustrate the effect that the energy spectrum of the beam has on the aerial image. **Figure 2–13** shows the fluence pattern produced when radiation is created at 50 kVp and at 70 kVp, with an appropriate decrease in mAs.

Note that the x-ray fluence penetrating the soft tissue is twice as great for the 70 kVp x rays as that produced at 50 kVp. Note also that the 70 kVp subject contrast in **Figure 2–13** is lower than the subject contrast at 50 kVp.

However, if the mAs were reduced for the 70 kVp beam to *one-half* its former value, the x-ray fluence emerging from both the soft tissue and the bone would also be *reduced by a factor of two*. Therefore, the subject contrast (ratio of fluences) would be unchanged.

Distance

The x-ray fluences in the aerial image can also be altered uniformly by moving the x-ray tube away from or toward the object. This can be demonstrated easily. In a darkened room, move a flashlight toward this printed page. The closer the light is to the book, the more brightly the page is illuminated. Exactly the same thing occurs with x rays.

As the distance from the object to the source of radiation is decreased, the x-ray fluence at the object increases. As the distance is increased, the radiation fluence at the object decreases. This results from the fact that both x rays and light travel in diverging straight lines, that is, they radiate from a point source. The relationship between distance and x-ray fluence is called the **inverse square law** because the radiation fluence varies inversely to the square of the distance from the source.

This effect is demonstrated in **Figure 2–14** in which the same x-radiation that covers a given area at distance D from the source disperses itself over four times as great an area at twice the distance, 2D (4 is the square of 2). This means that the radiation fluence at distance 2D from the target is one-fourth that at D. If a distance 3D were shown (three times the original one), the area covered by the radiation would be nine times that at distance D (the square of 3 is 9) and the fluence would be one-ninth that of D. An example of the inverse square law as it is applied in magnification technique imaging in the breast is given in Chapter 3, **Figure 3-12**.

A change in distance produces an effect similar to a change in mAs. In other words, subject contrast is unaffected by changes in distance. In order to produce radiographs of comparable overall blackening, *mAs must be increased to counteract the effect of increasing distance.*

It is important to note that when changing distance, consideration must be given to the effect this may have on image blur and on exposures in which a focused grid is used to reduce scattered radiation (grids are discussed in Chapter 3).

The amount by which the overall x-ray beam fluence is changed when mAs or distance is changed may be calculated arithmetically. See Appendix A.

Summary of Exposure Factors

1. Photon fluence of the aerial image is affected by mAs, spectrum, and distance.

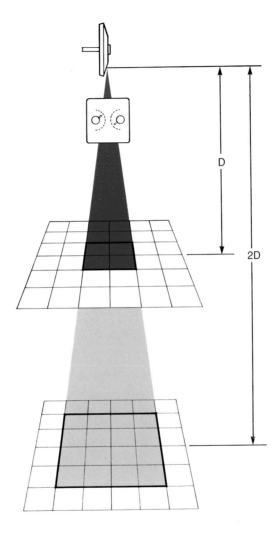

Figure 2–14 Inverse Square Law. As x rays travel farther from their source, their radiation fluence diminishes inversely as the square of the distance from the source.

2. When mAs or distance is used as a factor for the control of overall film blackening (optical density), subject contrast is not affected.

3. When the spectrum is altered, either by changing kVp, voltage waveform, or target-filter combination, both the overall optical density and the subject contrast are altered. Furthermore, filtering or hardening the x-ray spectrum increases the penetrating power of the beam but reduces subject contrast.

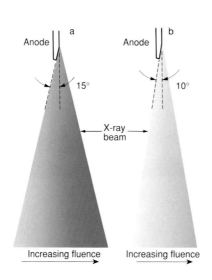

Figure 2–15 Heel Effect. (a and b) A variation in the fluence of the x-ray beam along the cathode-anode axis of the x-ray tube is known as the heel effect. X-ray fluence decreases toward the anode side of the x-ray beam. (b) The heel effect is more pronounced when using a steep-angle target tube.

HEEL EFFECT

It might be assumed that the fluence of x-radiation over the entire area covered by the beam entering the patient is constant. However, this is not entirely correct. Actually, there is a variation in photon fluence due to the angle at which the x rays emerge from within the target material.

This variation in fluence across the x-ray beam associated with the angle of x-ray emission from the focal spot is called the **heel effect**. As shown in **Figure 2–15**, the *x-ray fluence diminishes fairly rapidly from the central ray toward the anode side of the tube and increases slightly toward the cathode side.* Furthermore, the heel effect increases as the anode angle decreases. (See **Figure 1–18** and the discussion on line-focus principle in Chapter 1.)

Thoughtful use of the heel effect can produce radiographs with more balanced optical densities (film blackening) of body parts that differ in absorption. For example, in radiography of the thoracic vertebrae, the thinner cervical area should be exposed by the lower fluence (anode) side of the beam. Similarly, proper positioning of the x-ray tube allows radiation from the cathode side of the beam to expose the thicker mediastinal area. **Figure 2–16a** shows a lack of balance in optical densities because the cervical area was overexposed and the thorax underexposed due to incorrect alignment of the tube and the patient. By taking advantage of the heel effect and directing the higher fluence portion of the beam (cathode side) through the more absorbing mediastinal region, the radiograph will be improved **(Figure 2–16b)**. The effect of positioning the x-ray tube (cathode-anode

a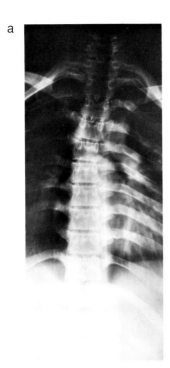

b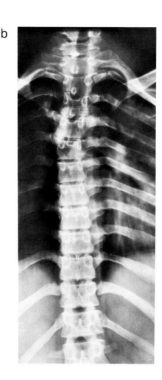

Figure 2–16 Radiographs Demonstrating the Heel Effect. **(a)** When the x-ray tube is positioned incorrectly with respect to the thoracic vertebrae of a patient, the cervical vertebrae will be overexposed and the thoracic vertebrae underexposed. Overexposure of the cervical area of the radiograph results when the portion of the x-ray beam with higher fluence (cathode end of the tube) is directed through the thinner, less absorbing structures of the cervical area. When the lower fluence portion of the beam (anode end of the tube) is directed through the thicker, lower thoracic area, underexposure results. **(b)** Radiographic optical densities can be balanced by positioning the anode portion of the beam towards the cervical area and the cathode portion towards the thicker thoracic area.

relationship) when imaging the pelvis is shown schematically in **Figure 2–17**.

Because the x-ray beam fluence is more uniform near the central ray, the heel effect is not a disadvantage when only the central portion of the beam is used. Furthermore, the heel effect is not a technical concern when focal spot-film distance (FFD) is increased, or when beam-limiting devices reduce the area of the x-ray beam, as when imaging a small anatomical area.

In this text, the term focal spot-film distance will be shortened to focal-film distance (FFD). **Figure 2–18** provides commonly used distance nomenclature and abbreviations.

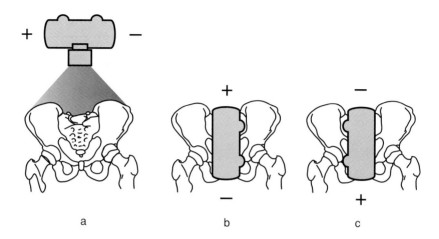

a   b   c

Figure 2–17 X-ray Tube Positioning to Minimize the Heel Effect. With the x-ray tube oriented transverse to the pelvis in the AP position, variations in optical density owing to the heel effect could occur. **(a)** The side of the pelvis imaged by the anode portion of the beam may exhibit less film blackening than the opposite side of the pelvis imaged by the cathode side of the beam. **(b)** If the x-ray tube were positioned with the cathode side of the tube towards the pubic area, these structures could be overexposed. **(c)** For an average-sized patient, when the tube is positioned with the cathode towards the thicker lumbosacral area and the anode towards the pubic area, a more evenly exposed radiograph is possible.

Distance Nomenclature			
FFD	Focal-film distance	SID	Source-image receptor distance
		SSD	Source-skin distance
FOD	Focal-object distance	SOD	Source-object distance
OFD	Object-film distance	OID	Object-image receptor distance

Figure 2–18 Distance Nomenclature. This text uses the terms focal-film and focal-object distance as abbreviated forms of focal spot-film and focal spot-object distances.

GEOMETRY OF IMAGE FORMATION

One goal of medical radiography is to obtain as accurate an image as possible. Two of the many factors that affect this accuracy are the *degree of blur* and the *size of the image*. A demonstration that you can perform yourself using light bulbs will illustrate these factors (**Figure 2–19**).

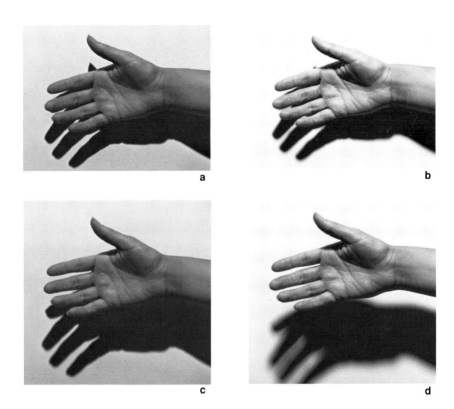

Figure 2–19 Effect of Source and Distance on Shadows. **(a)** When using a small light source with the hand close to the wall, a relatively sharp shadow is produced. **(b)** With the hand in the same position but with a large light source, some blurring of the shadow is observed. **(c)** With a small lamp and the hand moved away from the wall, the shadow enlarges and blurs. **(d)** With the hand in the same position using the large light source, the shadow becomes even more enlarged and blurred. In this analogy, a small (large) light source corresponds to a small (large) focal-spot size. The hand represents an object being radiographed at different object-film distances (OFD). The image on the wall represents the radiographic image.

Geometric Blur and Magnification

Obtain a small, clear lamp, such as a 7-watt night-light or small flashlight. Set it up about three feet from a wall, turn it on, and place your hand an inch or two from the wall. Notice that the shadow produced by this small light source is nearly the same size as your hand and that the edges are quite distinct (**Figure 2–19**). Now, move your hand away from the wall toward the light. Observe the manner in which the shadow grows larger and fuzzier along the edges. Next, substitute a large frosted bulb for the night-light and notice that the edge of the shadow is a little fuzzy even when your hand is close to the wall. The blur is

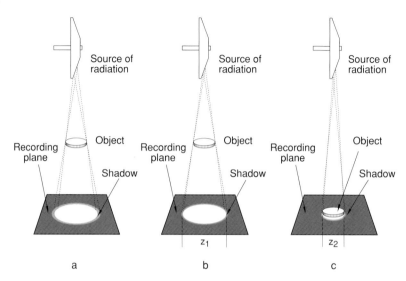

Figure 2–20 The Geometry of Image Formation. **(a)** Note the blurring of the radiographic image owing to a large focal spot, an increased object-film distance, and a decreased focal-object distance. **(b)** A smaller focal spot reduces image blur, Z_1. **(c)** The combination of a smaller focal spot, decreased object-film distance, and increased focal-object distance minimizes image blur, Z_2. This geometric combination minimizes object enlargement.

caused by the *larger* light source. Again, move your hand toward the lamp and see how the shadow enlarges and the blur increases.

Since the aerial x-ray image is also a shadow of the object, *these same principles of shadow formation apply to radiography*. Image blur and distortion may be minimized by using a smaller x-ray source (focal spot), reducing the object-film distance, and increasing the focal-object distance.

These points are illustrated in **Figure 2–20**. The *blur* of the radiographic image caused by a large focal spot and increased object-film distance, and a decreased focal-object distance is demonstrated **(Figure 2–20a)**. The improvement produced by reducing the size of the focal spot is shown, although the distances are unchanged **(Figure 2–20b)**. The optimal result is achieved by using a small focal spot, a decreased object-film distance, and an increased focal-object distance **(Figure 2–20c)**. The enlarged *image size* (Z_1) that results from the use of a long object-film distance and a short focal-object distance is also shown. Note the more accurate image size (Z_2) when the object is as close as possible to the image receptor and farther from the focal spot.

Distortion

Distortion is the enlargement of different parts of a structure by different

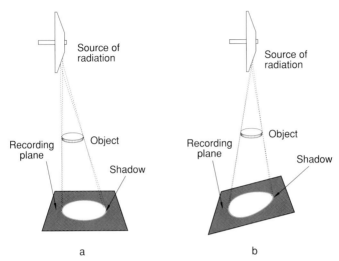

Figure 2–21 X-ray Source and Recording Plane Position. **(a)** Although the source of radiation is not vertically centered above the circular object, an approximately circular shadow is formed if the object and recording plane (image receptor) are parallel. **(b)** When the object and image receptor plane are not parallel, the object is distorted.

amounts. For example, if the focal spot is not centered with respect to the object, enlargement will occur and the shadow will not remain circular (**Figure 2–21**). In **Figure 2–20**, the object and recording surface are parallel and, accordingly, the circular objects appear as circular shadows. If they are not parallel, as in **Figure 2–21b**, the shadow will be distorted. In **Figure 2–21b**, the part of the shadow farther away from the object is enlarged more than the nearer part, making the circular object appear egg-shaped on the recording plane.

Magnification is a form of distortion where the shape of an object is not substantially altered. Magnification is rarely uniform, however. Objects farther from the image receptor will always be magnified more than objects closer to the image receptor, for the same FFD (other factors remaining unchanged).

Distortion (unequal enlargement) and magnification (fairly uniform enlargement) can sometimes be useful by making it easier to see structures that otherwise might be obscured. Note that there is minimal distortion of either object in **Figure 2–22**—both the objects and the shadows are circular. However, a change in the direction of the x-ray beam changes the relationship of the shadows (even though the relationship of the objects is unchanged).

In **Figure 2–22**, if one could see only the shadows and not the structures producing them (as is the case for internal anatomical structures in radiography), one might conclude that the shadow was produced by a single structure with a figure-eight shape. To determine that the shadow was comprised of more than

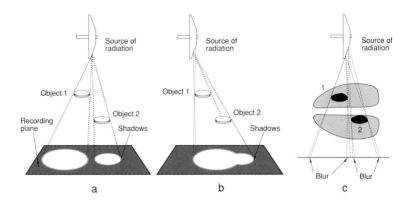

Figure 2–22 The Relationship of the X-ray Source to the Edges of Two Objects. When multiple objects are located in different planes, separate or overlapping shadows may occur. Objects 1 and 2 are separated in **(a)** but overlap in **(b)** due to their relationship to the source of radiation. **(c)** A schematic representation of the chest in the lateral position demonstrates distinct images of both objects, but with differences in blur and magnification owing to their relationships to the x-ray source and image receptor.

one structure, a second image from a different angle must be obtained.

In radiography, not only the shadow of the edge of an object, but all of the shadows of the structures within it are involved because x rays penetrate the object. The same principles apply to the shadows of internal structures as apply to edges. For instance, if one of these internal structures is farther away from the image receptor plane than another, the structure farther away will be less sharp and more magnified **(Figures 2–22 and 2–23)**. This information can be useful, for example, in establishing the position of a lesion.

Motion

Another factor that contributes to image blur is motion. Motion, either of the structures being radiographed, the exposing equipment, or the image receptor due to Bucky motion can cause severe blurring of the image. When possible, the part under examination should be immobilized. Exposure times should also be as short as necessary to minimize the blur caused by motion **(Figure 2–24)**.

Summary of Image Information

The geometry of image formation may be summarized by the following five rules for accurate image formation.

1. The focal spot should be as small as is practical, taking into account possible blooming effects (see Chapter 1).

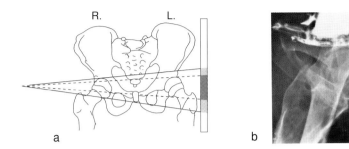

a   b

Figure 2–23 Unequal Magnification. A pelvis in the left lateral position demonstrates unequal magnification of the femurs. Note the projection of the right head of the femur (solid line) versus the left femoral head (dotted line). **(a)** A significant increase in size and image blur occurs with the right femoral head. **(b)** The image of the right femur, which is farther from the image receptor, demonstrates greater magnification and increased image blur when compared with the left femur, which is closer to the image receptor.

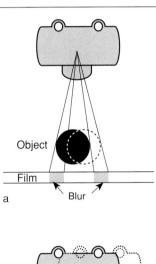

Figure 2–24 The Effect of Motion on Image Blur. Motion by either **(a)** the object under study or **(b)** the x-ray tube degrades the image by increasing image blur. **(c)** Patient motion seen while examining the cervical vertebrae in the AP position results in an unacceptable image.

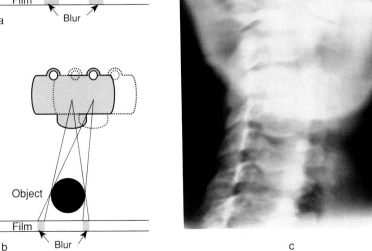

c

2. The object being radiographed should be as close as possible to the image receptor.

3. The distance between the object to be examined and the image receptor should be as small as is practical.

4. Generally speaking, the x-ray tube should be as nearly parallel to the image receptor as possible to record adjacent structures in their true spatial relationships.

5. As far as is practical, the plane of interest in the object should be parallel to the image receptor.

6. Efforts should be made to minimize voluntary and involuntary motion blur.

SUMMARY

A radiograph is an image created when objects in the x-ray beam absorb some, but not all, of the x-ray photons in the beam. Photons that penetrate the object and reach the image receptor cause blackening on the processed radiograph. X-ray photons that are absorbed do not reach the image receptor, producing clear areas on the processed radiograph that appear white when illuminated by a viewbox.

Differences in x-ray absorption produce the shades of gray that contain the information in a radiograph. These differences in absorption are caused by the spectrum of the x-ray beam and the characteristics of the absorbing material. The aerial image is the term used to describe the patterns of x-ray fluences incident on the image receptor.

Subject contrast is the ratio of photon fluence emerging from different parts of an object being radiographed. Subject contrast increases as differences in x-ray absorption increase.

Radiographs are subject to geometric blurring and magnification due to the finite size of the focal spot and the distance from the object to the image receptor. Motion of the patient or the x-ray tube also contributes to image blur.

Chapter 3
Scattered Radiation

The introductory discussions of x-ray absorption presented an idealized view of x-ray imaging. It was assumed that when an object was exposed to x-radiation, the x-ray photons were either absorbed by the object or passed through the object. It was also assumed that the only photons to reach the image receptor were those originating at the focal spot, traveling in a straight line, passing directly through the object, and terminating at the image receptor. These photons are collectively called **primary radiation**. While convenient and easy to visualize, this model does not take into account the significant effect of scattered radiation, and the resulting degradation of the image.

X-ray photons travel in straight lines when undisturbed. When an x-ray photon interacts with matter, it may simply be absorbed, or it may undergo a somewhat more complex interaction called **scattering**. In diagnostic medical radiography, scattering occurs when an x-ray photon interacts with an atom in its path in such a way as to cause the photon to lose some of its energy and to change its direction of travel. Another term often used to describe scattered radiation is **secondary radiation**.

EFFECT ON SUBJECT CONTRAST

If you have driven an automobile on a foggy night, you have probably experienced the effects of light scattering. On a clear night, light photons arising from the headlights of the car are reflected by an object in the road, for example, the white stripe in the center of the road. The surrounding pavement is dark and reflects very few light photons. Light receptors in your eyes detect the reflected photons from the white stripe, as well as the absence of reflected light from the dark pavement. The result is a clear, unambiguous high-contrast image of the road.

In the presence of fog, however, the water droplets scatter the light photons. Light photons produced at the headlight are scattered, reducing the number that reach the pavement. Light photons reflected by the white stripe undergo so many changes in direction that the eye is often unable to distinguish between the reflecting white stripe and the dark pavement. As a result, it is difficult to perceive the white stripe in the road. This example of image degradation due to scattering of light photons is analogous to the effect of scattered x-radiation in medical radiographic imaging.

When x-ray photons are scattered by interactions within the patient, the resulting change in their direction of travel produces an overall hazy appearance in the radiograph. **Figure 3–1** illustrates the effect of scattered radiation, and the reduction in scattered radiation obtained by the use of a beam-limiting device.

Some x-ray photons produced at the target are absorbed by the bone. Other photons are transmitted to the image receptor through the surrounding soft tissue. Consequently, the image receptor would be exposed to a relatively low photon fluence under the bone, and a higher fluence under the soft tissue. *Subject contrast*

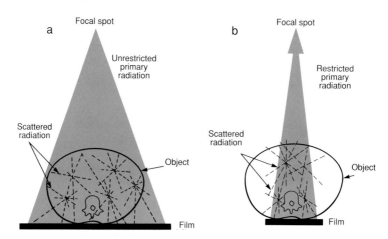

Figure 3–1 The Effect of a Beam-Limiting Device. **(a)** When the x-ray beam is not restricted, considerable scattered radiation is produced in a thick object. **(b)** When the volume irradiated by the beam is reduced, less scattered radiation is produced.

is defined as the ratio of photon fluences exiting regions of interest in a patient.* In the example of **Figure 3–2b**, the subject contrast between the bone and soft tissue is 100/20, or 5:1. Therefore, five times as many x-ray photons are available to expose the image receptor beyond the soft tissue as there are beyond the bone.

Figure 3–2c demonstrates the effect of scattered radiation on subject contrast. When scatter is produced in the patient, the exposed tissue regions become broad sources of x-radiation. Unlike the x-ray beam, which emanates from a tiny focal spot, scattered photons are produced over a large area, in fact, over the entire exposed region of the body. Because they are not produced by a point source, scattered radiation ultimately contributes little useful information to the image. It does, however, increase the photon fluence beyond both the bone and soft tissue regions of the thigh. In our example, consider the effect on subject contrast if the scattered radiation adds a uniform photon fluence of 20 to the bone and soft tissue regions of the thigh. With scatter, the subject contrast falls from 100/20 or 5:1 to 120/40 or 3:1. As shown, *the effect of scattered radiation upon subject contrast is dramatic.* The numerical values of subject contrast quantify the effect seen on radiographs. Images with excessive scattered radiation have a "foggy" appearance, diminishing our ability to differentiate objects.

Because of scatter, the exposed areas within the patient are themselves a source of unwanted radiation that can expose film. Furthermore, scattered radiation does

---

*Subject contrast does **not** refer to how black or how white areas are on x-ray film. This is a different concept, called *radiographic contrast*, which is discussed in Chapter 5.

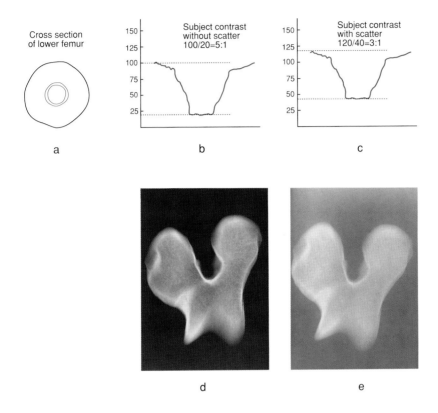

Figure 3–2 The Effect of Scatter on Subject Contrast. **(a)** Consider the aerial image produced during radiography of the lower femur. **(b)** In the absence of scatter, the subject contrast is high, 5:1. **(c)** Scatter is introduced, reducing the subject contrast to 3:1. **(d)** Representative radiograph made with a moderate kVp demonstrates excellent subject contrast. **(e)** When a higher kVp is used, scatter is increased and subject contrast is reduced.

not contribute to the formation of the useful image. On the contrary, it produces an overall x-ray fluence superimposed on the aerial image. The effect of this overlying fluence reduces subject contrast, that is, it decreases the ratio of x-ray fluences between neighboring structures in the aerial image.

SOURCES OF SCATTERED RADIATION

To control scattered radiation, it is necessary to understand the factors that govern its production. The factors that can be controlled are: kVp, field size, and the amount of tissue (for example, mass, thickness, and composition) being irradiated.

As an x-ray photon scatters, it loses some of its energy and changes direction.

After many scattering interactions, an individual photon loses so much of its energy that it can no longer emerge from the patient to "fog" the film. The higher the initial energy of the x-ray photon, the more possibilities for scatter, until the energy of the photon is exhausted. Therefore, *the use of a higher kVp beam will increase scatter production.*

The major source of scattered radiation is the irradiated segment of the patient; although scattered radiation may be produced by interactions between primary x-ray photons and *any* objects in their path. The amount of scattered radiation generated is related to the volume of matter irradiated—the larger the volume (generally the thicker the body part), the greater the scattered radiation, other factors remaining constant.

Concern for scatter arises primarily from its undesirable effect on subject contrast. It is usually more useful to know the *proportion* of scattered radiation in the beam that reaches the image receptor than the actual amount. In evaluating the effect of scatter on image quality, a useful quantity is the ratio of scattered photon fluence to primary photon fluence, called the *scatter-to-primary ratio*. In the case of heavy body parts, such as the abdomen, the fluence of scattered radiation may be 10 or more times as great as the primary image-forming radiation. For a chest examination, it is widely accepted that the average fluence of the scattered radiation reaching the image receptor is about equal to that of the primary radiation. However, the ratio of scatter-to-primary radiation depends on relationships among the structures being radiographed, as well as field size and kVp. For example, in a chest radiograph, scattered radiation represents a larger percentage of the total radiation behind the heart shadow than behind the lungs, because there is more tissue mass in the mediastinum to produce scatter compared with the lungs, which are mostly air-filled.

REDUCING SCATTERED RADIATION

Beam Limitation

Minimizing scattered radiation substantially improves image quality. A most important rule to remember is that *the primary beam should be confined to a size and shape that will only cover the region of diagnostic interest.* Areas of the patient that are not irradiated cannot contribute to scatter or to patient dosage. A positive beam limitation (PBL) device prohibits exposure, unless the x-ray beam is restricted to the size of the screen-film cassette in use. In addition, several manual devices are available that can be attached to the x-ray tube for the purpose of restricting the x-ray field, including diaphragms, cones, and variable-aperture, beam-limiting devices (**Figure 3–3**).

Beam-limiting devices are commonly but inaccurately referred to as collimators. (A collimator is actually a device for producing light rays that are

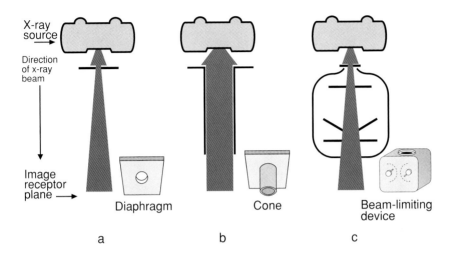

Figure 3–3 Beam-Limiting Devices. This illustration shows **(a)** an aperture diaphragm placed close to the x-ray source (target), **(b)** a cone with attached diaphragm, and **(c)** a variable-aperture, multiple-shutter, beam-limiting device. The lead shutter closest to the tube window in (c) reduces extra-focal radiation.

parallel to each other.) The rays emerging from these beam-limiting devices are not parallel as the word collimator suggests. They are divergent, that is, they travel in straight-line paths that spread farther away from one another with increasing distance from their source. In spite of this fact, variable-aperture, beam-limiting devices are usually referred to as collimators.

Aperture Diaphragms

Aperture diaphragms consist of sheets of lead with rectangular, square or circular openings **(Figure 3–3a)**. These are inserted into the x-ray beam near the window of the x-ray tube. They are usually used in conjunction with a cone or a variable-aperture, beam-limiting device.

Cones

Cones are metal tubes of various shapes and sizes **(Figure 3–3b)**. Some cones provide circular fields, others rectangular fields. The length of the cone, as well as the size of its opening, will affect the size of the x-ray field. Most dental x-ray equipment utilizes cones.

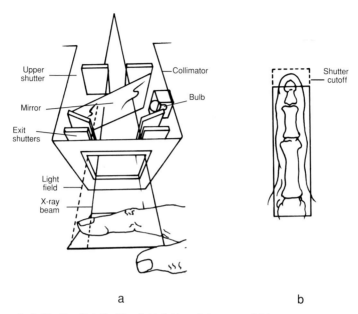

a   b

Figure 3–4 Shutter Cutoff. The light field and the x-ray field are only coincident when all shutters, the light bulb, and the mirror are properly aligned. Visualization of the light-field size is determined by the position of the exit shutters of the collimator. If an x-ray shutter nearer to the source is out of alignment, shutter cutoff of the x-ray beam may occur, particularly on a small field image. **(a)** The misaligned light beam and x-ray field are represented. **(b)** The resulting shutter cutoff is seen at the distal end of the finger.

Variable-Aperture, Beam-Limiting Devices

Variable-aperture, beam-limiting devices contain lead plates or shutters that can be adjusted to alter the size of the beam **(Figure 3–3c)**. In some of these devices, the shutters are positioned manually by adjusting indicator knobs that limit the x-ray field to the cassette size in use. More sophisticated devices use sensors, which detect the size of the cassette in use and automatically adjust the shutters to the size of the image receptor. (Further reduction in field size is possible by overriding the PBL system.) The variable-aperture, beam-limiting device usually contains cross hairs, a light-source, and a mirror to project the center and the outline of the x-ray field defined by the shutters onto the patient.

The "collimator" light bulb and the exit shutters form the light field that is seen on the patient. Only with proper adjustment of the light source and all shutters does this light field represent the actual x-ray field **(Figure 3–4)**.

Grids

Thick, heavy body parts, such as the abdomen, produce a much higher propor-

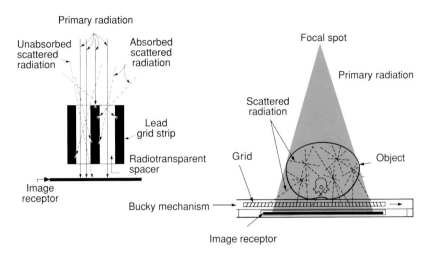

Figure 3–5 Cross Section of a Grid. **(Left)** A diagram of a small section of a grid showing how a large portion of the scattered radiation is absorbed and primary radiation passes through to the image detector. A single lead strip is shown as a complete absorber. In an actual grid, scattered rays may pass through several lead strips before being completely absorbed. **(Right)** A Bucky mechanism with a focused grid being moved towards the right is shown.

tion of scattered radiation than do thin parts, such as the hand. Therefore, high-quality images of many body parts require other means of controlling scattered radiation in addition to beam-limiting devices. A very effective mechanism for this purpose is called a grid **(Figure 3–5)**.

A **grid** is a device composed of alternating strips of lead and spacer material, bearing some resemblance to venetian blinds. A spacer material with low x-ray absorption characteristics is selected, usually fiber or aluminum. The alternating absorbent strips and spacer material are encased in a protective covering to provide strength and durability. As shown in **Figure 3–5**, the lead strips absorb a considerable amount of the oblique scattered radiation, that is, the photons not traveling in the direction of the primary beam. They also absorb some of the primary radiation. The spacers, which are *radiolucent,* allow most of the primary x-ray photons of the aerial image to pass through to the film.

Grid Ratio

The ratio of the height of the lead strips to the width of the radiolucent spacers is the **grid ratio**. For example, if the height of the lead strip is 8 times the width of the interspace, the grid ratio is 8:1; if the height is 16 times the width, the ratio is 16:1. Other factors held constant, the greater the ratio, the more efficiently the grid absorbs scattered radiation. The compromise, however, is that more primary radiation is also absorbed in a higher ratio grid. High-ratio grids require careful positioning of the x-ray tube to avoid cutoff.

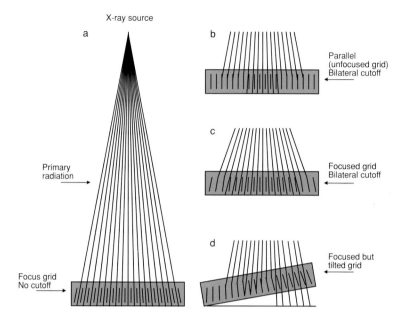

Figure 3–6 Grid Cutoff. **(a)** A grid must be centered beneath and perpendicular to the central ray of the x-ray tube. The tube must be positioned within the focal range recommended by the manufacturer. Under these conditions, primary radiation travels approximately parallel to the lead strips. Consequently, the x-ray fluence transmitted by the grid is uniform and there is no grid cutoff. **(b)** The lead strips in a parallel grid do not follow the divergent pattern of the x-ray beam. This causes progressively increasing misalignment of the lead strips toward the lateral aspects of the image. The transmitted x-ray fluence is decreased toward the edges of the grid, causing bilateral grid cutoff in the radiograph. **(c)** If the source-grid distance is not within the recommended focal range, the lead strips do not follow the divergent pattern of the x-ray beam. This causes bilateral grid cutoff toward the edges of the radiograph. **(d)** When a grid is not aligned perpendicular to the central ray of the x-ray beam, the lead strips do not follow the divergent pattern of the x-ray beam. This produces a non-uniform distribution of fluence beyond the grid, and grid cutoff in the radiograph.

Grid Focus and Cutoff

In an **unfocused grid**, the lead strips are parallel to one another **(Figure 3–6b)**, whereas a **focused grid** utilizes lead strips that are progressively angled so that lines extended from each strip converge to a point **(Figure 3–6a)**. The distance from this point of convergence, or **focal point**, to the grid is called its **focal distance**. *Ideally, the placement of the focal spot of the x-ray tube should coincide with the focal point of the grid.* In addition, the *central ray* of the beam should intersect the center of the grid perpendicularly for general radiography applications.

Focused grids usually have a **focal range** specified by the manufacturer, that is, a range of distances throughout which the grid can be satisfactorily used. If a

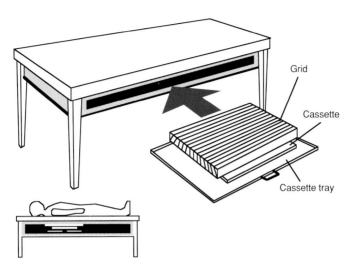

Figure 3–7 Position of a Grid in a Bucky Mechanism. The lead strips of a focused grid are shown with the protective outside cover removed. When the grid is installed in the Bucky mechanism, the strips are positioned parallel to the length of the table. This permits tilting of the x-ray tube parallel to the long dimension of the table without producing grid cutoff. A cassette in position in the cassette tray is shown beneath the grid.

grid is used outside its focal range, *bilateral cutoff* is observed **(Figure 3–6c)**. **Grid cutoff** is a progressive decrease in transmitted x-ray fluence toward the lateral aspects of the image. This is caused by the increasing misalignment of the lead strips and primary beam toward the sides of the grid. Shadows of the lead strips cast by the primary beam become wider, resulting in bilateral cutoff of the primary beam.

Cutoff can also be caused by improper centering of the x-ray tube over the grid (lateral decentering) or by tilting the tube laterally across the lead strips **(Figure 3–6d)**. However, the tube may be tilted longitudinally along the length of the strips without causing cutoff because the x rays remain parallel to the lead strips. Grids are designed for insertion into *Bucky mechanisms* so that the lead strips run parallel to the length of the table **(Figure 3–7)**. In this way, the x-ray tube may be tilted parallel to the long dimension of the table without producing grid cutoff.

Cutoff caused by a tilted grid is a common problem in mobile radiography. For this reason, low-ratio grids that offer more latitude in positioning are often used for portable radiography.

Figure 3–8 provides focal ranges for specified grid ratios that can be used without resulting in cutoff.

Parallel (unfocused) grids tend to produce cutoff **(Figure 3–6b)** unless used with small field sizes or at very long distances from the x-ray tube.

Bucky Mechanism – 40 in. FFD Focal Range	
Grid ratio	Focal range (in.)
5:1	28–72
8:1	34–44
12:1	36–40
16:1	40

Figure 3–8 Typical Grid Focal Ranges for a Bucky Mechanism

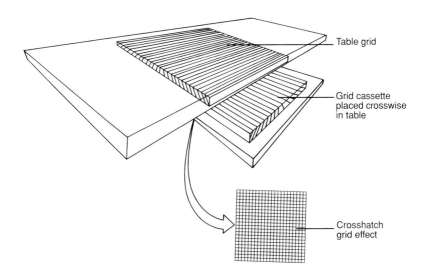

Figure 3–9 Crosshatch Grid. When examining a large patient, a lower ratio grid may not be adequate to minimize scatter. A grid cassette can be placed in the Bucky tray with its grid lines positioned at a right angle to the table grid, essentially forming a crosshatch grid.

For increased scatter reduction, crossed, crisscross or crosshatch grids may be used. They are essentially made from two linear grids one on top of the other, with lead strips perpendicular to one another. A grid cassette can be inserted crosswise into a conventional Bucky tray when a higher ratio grid is needed **(Figure 3–9)**.

Stationary vs Moving Grids

A stationary crosshatch grid was described by Dr. Gustav Bucky in 1913. With stationary grids, shadows of the lead strips are superimposed on the useful image. These "grid lines" may be tolerable in a radiograph when using a grid

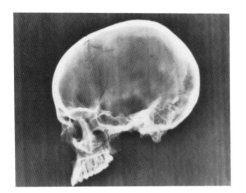

Figure 3–10 Grid Striping. Radiograph of a skull phantom showing light and dark bands (stripes) resulting from a very short exposure time. The dark stripes represent areas under the moving grid interspaces where the transmitted x-ray fluence was high. The light stripes represent areas under the moving lead strips where the transmitted x-ray fluence was low. If the exposure time had been longer, the areas covered by the interspaces and lead strips would be overlapped. This would have produced a more uniform distribution of x-ray fluence exiting the grid, and would have eliminated the striping effect in the image.

with very thin, uniformly spaced strips. In these cases, the very fine lines are not objectionable in the image, but are detectable upon close inspection.

Dr. Hollis E. Potter showed in 1920 that the pattern of the stationary crosshatch grid could be eliminated by using a grid made up of strips parallel to the length of the table, which moved perpendicular to the table during an exposure **(Figure 3–7)**. The motion blurs the grid lines and makes them indistinguishable on the radiograph. The device comprising a grid and the mechanism for moving it is called a **Potter-Bucky diaphragm**. Optimal use of a moving grid requires attention to the following technical details.

1. When a single-phase generator is used, the speed of the moving grid must be such that motion of the lead strips is not synchronized with the pulses of the x-ray machine, otherwise the strips will be imaged.

2. On the other hand, motion must be fast enough for a number of strips to pass a given point on the film during the exposure, or blurring will not be sufficient. Reciprocating mechanisms that move the grid back and forth are most commonly used.

3. The exposure time used must not be too short or the grid may not be able to move far enough to avoid producing a striped pattern or an irregular density pattern on the film **(Figure 3–10)**. These patterns arise from slight non-uniformities in the grid.

4. Equipment incorporating a Bucky diaphragm should be designed and maintained to minimize vibration and the resulting image blur.

5. Due to the size of the grid mechanism, the distance between patient and film is increased when using a Bucky diaphragm, thereby increasing the geometric blur and magnification in the image.

Line Spacing

Another factor that affects the efficiency of the grid in reducing scattered radiation is the number of lead strips or lines per centimeter or inch. This number may vary from 60 to 100 or more lines per inch, depending upon the application and the manufacturer. Grids with many thin lead strips per inch (100 or more) are often chosen for stationary use because the thinner strips are less visible in the radiograph.

Effect on Exposure

The grid absorbs a large part of the scattered radiation, as well as some of the primary radiation. It should be emphasized that scattered radiation adds no useful diagnostic information to the image. All x-radiation reaching the image receptor, including scattered radiation, contributes to film blackening. Therefore, when using a grid, radiation exposure (radiographic technique) must be increased (to compensate for this absorption) if we wish to avoid producing a radiograph that has less scatter but is underexposed. The required increase in radiographic technique depends on the efficiency of the grid in absorbing scattered radiation. The more efficient the grid, the greater the increase in technique factors. The increase also depends on the ratio of scattered to primary radiation, that is, upon the body part being radiographed.

Air Gap

An alternative to the grid technique for scatter reduction is the use of an air gap between the patient and the image receptor during an x-ray exposure. Recall that primary radiation travels in straight lines from the x-ray target to the image receptor, while scattered radiation originates within the patient and travels at many different angles to the primary radiation. When the patient is positioned in close proximity to the image receptor, much of the emerging scattered radiation reaches the receptor. When the patient is moved away from the detector, scattered photons tend to diverge much more rapidly than primary photons, due to their increased angle of trajectory (**Figure 3–11**). As a result, the proportion of scattered radiation reaching the image receptor is reduced.

Compromises in the use of the air gap technique take the form of image blur, magnification, and increased dose. As the air gap is increased, the size of the image is increased, always producing a magnified image. At the same time, images made using magnification technique always benefit from increased subject contrast due to the scatter reduction caused by the air gap.

To introduce the air gap, the patient must be moved closer to the x-ray tube, while the image receptor remains at a fixed distance from the x-ray tube. An alternative is to move the image receptor farther away from the patient, with the patient position held constant. In both cases, the **Entrance Skin Exposure (ESE)** to the patient is increased, compared with the ESE from a conventional grid (non-magnification) technique for an equally well-exposed radiograph.

If the patient is moved closer to the x-ray source, the reduced distance produces an increase in ESE due to the effect of the *inverse square law.* Conversely, radiation exposure decreases with distance from a point source of

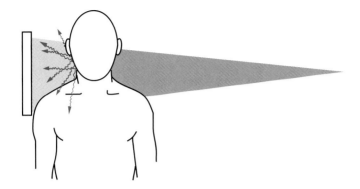

Figure 3–11 Air Gap Technique. An air gap (increased object-film distance) can be substituted for a grid to minimize the scattered radiation reaching the image receptor. Photons scattered at angles from the primary beam (red) diverge and often miss the image receptor due to the air gap. An increased focal-film distance minimizes the magnification associated with an increased object-film distance when examining the cervical spine in the lateral position.

radiation. The magnitude of the decrease is related to the square of the distance from the source. Consider this effect as it applies to **magnification imaging technique** in the breast. Assume an ESE to the breast of 1000 mR is required for a well-exposed radiograph using a grid (non-magnification) technique. This might correspond to machine factors of 26 kVp and 50 mAs **(Figure 3–12)**. The distance from the focal spot to the skin is equal to the FFD minus the compressed breast thickness minus the air gap, if any: 65 cm – 4 cm – 0 cm = 61 cm. For a 1.5X magnification, the distance from the focal spot to the entrance skin of the breast will be 65 cm – 4 cm – 22 cm = 39 cm. Since the breast is moved closer to the x-ray tube for the magnification technique than for the grid technique, the ESE will increase. The ESE for the breast positioned for a magnification view would be:

$$1000 \text{ mR } (61/39)^2 = 2450 \text{ mR}.$$

As previously discussed, the air gap employed in magnification technique is an excellent scatter reduction technique, eliminating the need for a grid to perform this function. Since a grid is not used, the mAs (and therefore ESE) may be reduced by about 50% (the Bucky factor) to produce a well-exposed radiograph, making the ESE about 1200 mR.

An understanding of the inverse square law and the Bucky factor permits us to calculate the radiation exposure and technique factors required to produce well-exposed radiographs at different distances. If the patient position is held constant and the image receptor moved farther away from the x-ray source (as with fluoroscopy, fluoro-spot filming or cineradiography), the primary radiation must

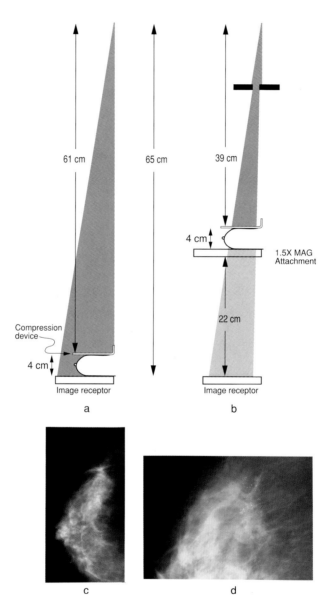

Figure 3–12 Magnification Technique in Mammography. **(a)** In a conventional mammographic image, the compressed breast is in close contact with the image receptor. **(b)** In magnification technique, the breast is positioned on a platform closer to the x-ray tube. **(c)** A conventional mammogram suggests pathology. **(d)** Improved visualization of this pathology through the use of magnification technique is shown. (Breast radiographs courtesy of Wende Logan-Young, M.D., Elizabeth Wende Breast Clinic, Rochester, New York.)

travel a greater distance. Here, the inverse square law predicts a dose reduction *at the image receptor*. To produce a comparably exposed radiograph, the tube output must be increased to compensate for the increased distance, thereby increasing the dose to the patient.

The technical requirements of the exam, coupled with the nature and amount of scatter produced, determine whether grid or air-gap technique is preferred for scatter reduction in a given exam. The air-gap technique is only used for selected imaging procedures. Air gap chest radiography, the lateral projection of the cervical spine, and direct enlargement techniques, such as in mammography and angiography, benefit from the scatter reduction provided by the air-gap technique. Because of the accentuated geometric blur inherent in magnified images, a smaller focal-spot size must be used than the focal-spot size used for conventional techniques. In both cases, scatter is reduced and subject contrast improved, at the cost of increased dose (ESE). Furthermore, smaller focal spots cannot tolerate the same heat as larger focal spots, resulting in limited mA for magnification technique.

Compression

Compressing a body part, for example, an obese abdomen, during an exam offers the following benefits.

1. *Increased subject contrast.* The volume of tissue irradiated is decreased when compressed due to displacement of tissue sideways out of the beam as pressure is applied. This reduces the proportion of scattered radiation and increases subject contrast.

2. *Reduced image blur from motion.* The body part is less likely to move when compressed and therefore the possibility of increased blur owing to motion is reduced.

3. *Reduced geometric blur.* Structures of interest are pressed closer to the image receptor, thereby reducing geometric blur **(Figure 2-20)**.

4. *Reduced patient dose.* A thinner body part requires less radiation exposure to produce a well-exposed radiograph.

In mammography, compression must be used to improve image quality and reduce dosage. Subject contrast is increased, image blur owing to motion is reduced, and geometric blur is reduced by bringing structures within the breast closer to the image receptor. Unlike other compression techniques, in breast compression, the actual volume of tissue irradiated remains constant. However, by reducing the breast thickness, there are fewer opportunities for multiple scattering events. Additional scatter reduction can be achieved by using the magnification technique with *spot compression*. In this case, irradiated tissue volume is reduced, since only a small, well-compressed segment of the breast is exposed.

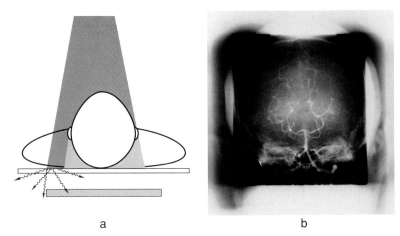

a   b

Figure 3–13 Image Undercutting Due to a Primary Beam Leak. **(a)** A projection of the skull demonstrates a primary beam leak. The unattenuated primary beam strikes the tabletop producing scatter (red), which results in unacceptable blackening of portions of the edges of the skull image. **(b)** Note the excessive film blackening (due to undercutting) on the image in the areas where a primary beam leak has occurred. The extraneous details surrounding the primary field of view are due to extra-focal radiation; see **Figure 3-14**.

Backscatter

For most medical radiography, the part of the patient irradiated is the principal source of scattered radiation. However, other materials in the x-ray beam, such as the table and cassette tray, also act as sources of scattered radiation. Radiation arising from such sources behind the image plane may be scattered back to the image; this is sometimes referred to as **backscatter**. Limiting the size of the x-ray beam so that it does not exceed the area of the image receptor is the most effective way of reducing backscatter. Most cassettes contain lead-foil backing to prevent backscatter from reaching the image receptor.

Undercutting

The shape of such body parts as the skull, shoulder or abdomen cause a portion of the x-ray beam to extend beyond the edge of the part being examined. The fluence of this portion of the beam is high relative to adjacent areas, where it has been partially absorbed in the body. Consequently, considerable scattered radiation may be generated in the tabletop and other material irradiated by the unattenuated beam. This scattered radiation produces an undesirable effect sometimes referred to as **undercutting**, which reduces subject contrast primarily along the periphery of the body part. Undercutting reduces peripheral contrast of the image by excessively

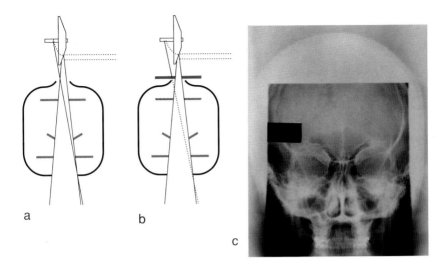

Figure 3–14   Extra-Focal Radiation.   When electrons rebound from the target and strike metallic areas other than the actual focal spot, additional sources of radiation occur. **(a)** These x-ray photons produce an unwanted image of the object outside of the primary field of view. **(b)** The introduction of a lead insert (red) as close as possible to the window of the x-ray tube considerably reduces the contribution of extra-focal radiation. **(c)** A tightly collimated skull radiograph demonstrates the effect of extra-focal radiation, represented by an ill-defined image of the outline of the skull. The black rectangle on the right side of the skull masks the identity of the patient or radiographer.

darkening the image. This problem can be lessened by placing shielding material, such as lead rubber, alongside the body part to absorb the unattenuated x–ray beam, thereby effectively reducing undercutting **(Figure 3–13)**. Compensation filters at or near the collimator exit also help minimize undercutting.

EXTRA-FOCAL RADIATION

Extra-focal or **off-focus radiation** is x-radiation emitted from parts of the x-ray tube other than the target **(Figure 3–14)**. Extra-focal radiation degrades image quality and its effect is therefore commonly misinterpreted as a result of scatter. Unlike scattered radiation, it does not arise from interaction of the primary beam with the patient. Extra-focal radiation is produced in the x-ray tube when improperly focused electrons interact with material outside the focal spot. Because the x rays produced by these electrons radiate in all directions, they extend beyond the borders of the primary beam defined by beam-limiting devices, and add an overall photon fluence to the aerial image. As in the case of scatter, the addition of this overlying photon fluence reduces subject contrast.

Several methods are available for reducing extra-focal radiation. A fixed or variable-aperture diaphragm may be inserted as close as possible to the focal spot (**Figure 3–14**). An alternative is to use a tube with a tungsten-alloy target ring embedded in a graphite (carbon) anode to reduce extra-focal radiation. Instead of the glass envelope and glass window of most x-ray tubes, mammography x-ray tubes use a metal case (with a beryllium window) operated at ground potential. This technique draws improperly focused electrons to the x-ray tube wall, effectively minimizing the production of extra-focal radiation in the vicinity of the target.

SUMMARY

When an x-ray photon interacts with matter, it may be absorbed, transmitted unaffected or scattered. Scattered x-ray photons have less energy than their parent *primary* photons and are produced at different angles from the primary beam. Scatter reduces subject contrast in the same way that fog impairs our ability to see while driving on a damp night. Scatter can be reduced by the use of beam limitation, grids, air-gap technique, and compression. Unlike scattered radiation, which arises from the patient, extra-focal radiation is produced when electrons interact with matter *outside* the focal spot.

Chapter 4

Recording the Image– Intensifying Screens

Up to this point, the discussion has been concerned primarily with factors that affect the aerial image, that is, the invisible distribution of x-ray fluences emerging from the object being radiographed. In conventional radiography, the image receptor, which consists of intensifying screens and x-ray film, converts the invisible information of the aerial image into a physical format that can be seen and interpreted.

CHARACTERISTICS OF IMAGE RECEPTORS

The purpose of the image receptor is to *absorb* the x-ray photons in the aerial image, to convert this information into a *display* format, and often to provide a permanent archival record of the information for future reference. Some important characteristics of an ideal image receptor include:

1. **Spatial Fidelity.** The image receptor must faithfully reproduce the information in the aerial image to which it is exposed **(Figure 4–1)**. Sharp edges, smooth curves, and fine detail must be accurately reproduced and displayed, without introducing *artifacts* that distract the attention of the observer.

2. **Amplification.** To the extent that an image receptor can amplify the information in the aerial image without compromising spatial fidelity, a high-quality radiograph may be produced using the least amount of radiation exposure, consistent with image quality requirements. Intensifying screens have virtually replaced direct exposure imaging. The amplification provided by screens results in reduced dosage and associated benefits without compromising overall image quality.

3. **Logistical Considerations.** An ideal image receptor is convenient to handle, view, compare with other diagnostic results from other imaging modalities, and store. These important human factors are often overlooked in evaluating image receptors.

4. **Cost.** Quality products must be used that do not burden the health care system with excessive costs.

5. **Environmental Effects.** All components involved in the life cycle of an image receptor must produce minimal negative impact on the environment.

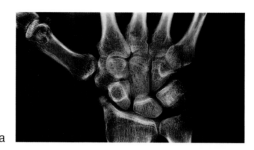

a

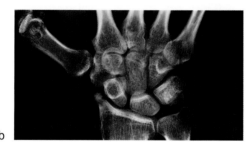

b

Figure 4-1 Image Blur. Representative radiograph of the carpal bones of the wrist. **(a)** A small focal spot was used to minimize image blur. **(b)** This wrist image was deliberately blurred photographically to simulate the effect of a large focal spot, which produces increased image blur.[4]

The first medical radiographic image receptors consisted of a silver-halide coating on a glass plate **(Figure 4–2)**. Such plates served all of the functions of the image receptor. They absorbed the information in the aerial image, converted the x-ray information into a visible image, and presented the image for handling, viewing, and archival storage.

Subsequent efforts to improve medical radiographic imaging were therefore directed at separating the functions of the image receptor into distinct components. Film was already available and was designed primarily to absorb visible light and to display high-quality images.

The most identifiable characteristic of x-radiation is its ability to penetrate matter. The high energy of x-ray photons and the penetrating power of x-radiation leads to both their unique usefulness in medical imaging and the difficulties encountered in capturing and displaying the information contained in an x-ray beam.

For example, of the x-ray fluence in the primary beam emerging from a patient, only about 1% or 2% is absorbed by a sheet of x-ray film (direct exposure), while 98% or more passes directly through the film and does not contribute to the image.

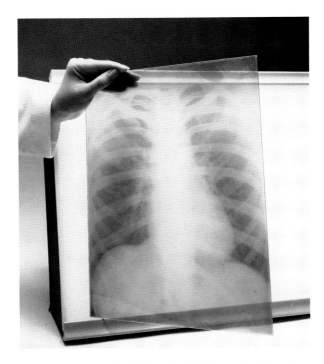

Figure 4–2 Glass Plate Radiograph. Prior to the 1920's, most radiographs were made on single-emulsion glass plates. This radiograph of the chest was made in 1912.[5]

Early medical radiographers recognized the advantages in using more of this wasted x-ray energy.

The **intensifying screen** was designed to optimize absorption of x-radiation and to convert absorbed x-ray energy into visible light, which would then be absorbed by the film. The introduction of fluorescent intensifying screens significantly altered the course of medical radiographic imaging. It led to the coating of photosensitive emulsion on both sides of the x-ray film, doubling the light absorption of the single-coated material.

An intensifying screen (often simply called a screen) is the sheet of material that is attached with a double-sided tape to the inside of an x-ray cassette. A **cassette** is a light-tight holder for the screen and the film, which keeps them in close contact. A screen contains a layer of phosphors, along with other components that optimize its performance. (Screen structure is covered in more detail later in this chapter.)

Screen-film image receptors are by no means the only image detectors in

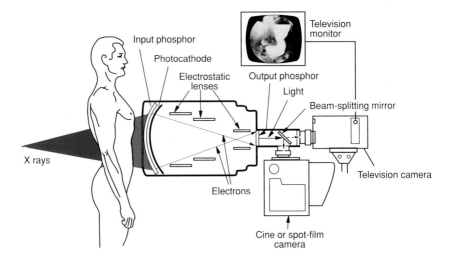

Figure 4–3 Image Intensifier System. X rays emerging from the patient are converted to light in the input phosphor. The light emitted from this fluorescent layer causes electrons to be given off by the photocathode. The electrons are accelerated and focused by an electrostatic field onto the output phosphor to produce a minified fluorescent image of the original x-ray pattern. The image on the output phosphor is much brighter but considerably smaller than that of the input phosphor. This image can be viewed directly or through closed-circuit television. It also can be photographed by cine or spot-film cameras.

common use today. **Image intensifier tubes** convert the x-ray aerial image to a visible light image on the tube's output phosphor. Traditionally, the image on the output phosphor of the image intensifier is directly imaged onto film, rapidly transported in roll form (cineradiography or 70 mm to 105 mm film) or cut-film (100 mm film) to provide images of dynamic events within the patient **(Figure 4–3)**. These brilliant light images can be captured by a video camera, similar in principle to a home video camcorder. The output of the video camera may be directly displayed on an analog video fluorography system, or digitized and used to produce digital fluoroscopic images, which can be manipulated by a computer. In addition, **storage phosphors** emit light in response to any x-ray exposure and can store the information in the aerial image for later *read out* and display. These imaging methods will be discussed in more detail in Chapter 8.

FLUORESCENT INTENSIFYING SCREENS

The Law of Conservation of Energy requires that all of the energy entering a small region must also leave that region. When high-energy x-ray photons encounter any substance, the photons will be absorbed, scattered or pass through unaffected. Substances called *phosphors* can absorb high-energy x-ray photons and re-emit this energy as many lower energy *light photons*. This process, known as **fluorescence**, occurs in an *intensifying screen* when each high-energy x-ray photon is converted by the phosphor into many thousands of lower energy light photons. In this way, the screen acts as an image amplifier, converting the aerial image, which is made up of relatively few x-ray photons, into an image made up of many thousands of times more light photons.

Kinds of Phosphors

Prior to the invention of the image intensifier tube, it was customary for radiologists to study body parts in motion by fluoroscopy. Fluoroscopy required a completely darkened room. After dark-adaptation of the eyes, the x-ray tube was energized, producing a lengthy x-ray exposure to the patient, the screen, and the fluoroscopist. The fluoroscopist looked directly at the moving images produced on a fluorescent screen that was exposed to the aerial image of the patient. These viewing screens contained a zinc sulfide phosphor that emitted yellow-green light. This phosphor was chosen because the human eye is most sensitive to light of this color. Fluorescent calcium tungstate ($CaWO_4$) intensifying screens and radiographic film followed for use in "still" radiographic imaging, to obtain an image in a shorter time and with less exposure than was possible with x-ray film alone. Calcium tungstate was chosen because it emits photons in the ultraviolet and blue regions of the electromagnetic spectrum. Silver-halide emulsions used in x-ray film are very sensitive to light photons in this energy range (color). More recently, phosphors such as barium sulfate, barium fluorochloride, lanthanum oxybromide, and oxysulfides of the rare-earth elements (gadolinium, lanthanum, and yttrium) have been used in intensifying screens.

Phosphor Characteristics

For a phosphor to be suitable for use in intensifying screens, it must meet certain requirements. Some of these are:
• high x-ray absorption,
• high conversion efficiency (that is, efficient conversion of x-ray photons to light photons),
• a light emission spectrum appropriate for use with film,
• suitability for manufacture,
• tolerance of a variety of ambient conditions, such as tropical heat and humidity, and
• freedom from *afterglow* and from delay in brightness *buildup*.

The term *fluorescence* is used to describe phosphor emissions that occur relatively soon after absorption of the x-ray photon. **Phosphorescence** or **after-**

glow is the characteristic of a phosphor to continue to give off light after the x-ray exposure has ceased. If this glow continues for more than a small fraction of a second, there may be interference with successive images, for example, as when x-ray exposures are made in rapid succession with serial film changers.

Buildup refers to the time required for the phosphor crystal to reach maximum brightness after an x-ray absorption event occurs. In most phosphors, this is so rapid that it is of no practical concern.

The requirements listed previously suggest some characteristics that should be optimized in designing or selecting intensifying screens. Understanding of these characteristics has led to improvements, such as the production of screens made from the lanthanide (rare-earth) series of elements. To illustrate, at 85 kVp, a pair of gadolinium oxysulfide (rare-earth) screens absorbs about 50% more x-ray photons than does a pair of calcium tungstate screens of the same thickness. The phosphor crystals in gadolinium oxysulfide screens also generate more than three times as much light as do those in calcium tungstate screens for each x-ray photon absorbed. Rare-earth screens permit a significant reduction in x-ray exposure (relative to that required for calcium tungstate screens of the same thickness) without increasing image blur. The amount of exposure reduction depends on many factors, including the kVp used to make the exposure.

Green-Emitting Screens

Some rare-earth phosphors emit a large part of their light in the green region of the visible light spectrum. Orthochromatic films, which are particularly sensitive to green light, take advantage of this light output. Such films are sometimes referred to as "green-sensitive," even though they are also sensitive to blue and ultraviolet radiation.

Intensification

Each time a phosphor crystal absorbs an x-ray photon, it emits a flash of light consisting of many light photons. Thousands of these flashes occur in each square millimeter of the screen during exposure. The brightness of this emitted light relates to the x-ray energy deposited in that minute portion of the screen. The greater the absorbed x-ray fluence, the greater the brightness of the emitted light. Therefore, over the entire surface of the screen, differences in absorbed x-ray fluence are transformed into differences in the brightness of light emitted.

X-ray film, which is highly sensitive to these visible light photons, captures the transient light image for viewing and archival storage. Silver halide emulsion is the essential component of x-ray film. While particularly well-suited to recording a light image, silver halide emulsion is a notably poor absorber of x-radiation.

Intensifying screens are a separate component of the imaging system. They are specifically designed to optimize the absorption of x rays and their conversion to light energy. The absorption of one x-ray photon results in the emission of thousands of light photons from the screen.

It is common to limit our use of the term *amplifier* to electronic devices, such as audio amplifiers, which increase the volume of sound. Electronic video amplifiers are used to increase the brightness and contrast of video signals, for example, from a TV signal captured in an antenna or from a cable connection. In this respect, it is acceptable to apply the term "image amplifier" to the screen-film image receptor, which increases the relatively fewer number of x-ray photons in the aerial image to a much higher number of light photons for absorption and display on processed radiographic film.

Light photons emitted by the screen are more readily absorbed by the film than are the more energetic x-ray photons, most of which pass through the film. The image receptor combines an intensifying screen with a spectrally (color) matched* light-sensitive film. The result is higher x-ray absorption, greater conversion to light, and more effective use of the resulting light by the spectrally matched film. This more efficient use of the x-radiation in the aerial image permits patient radiation exposure to be reduced by factors of 10 to 100 times or more, relative to that required for a direct exposure technique made without screens. The intensification, or **intensifying factor**, is used to define the radiation exposure required *without* screens divided by the exposure required *with* screens to provide the same film blackening effect. The intensification factor depends on the type of screen and film used, as well as on exposure factors, such as kilovoltage and type of examination.

Some of the advantages offered by intensification and the resulting reduction in radiation exposure are:

• reduced radiation exposure to patients and personnel,
• shorter exposure times, thereby decreasing image blur from patient motion,
• decreased heat production in the x-ray tube due to shorter exposures or lower mA values,
• increased flexibility in choice of kVp, which allows adjustment of subject contrast, and
• decreased focal-spot size to minimize geometric blur and to improve magnification x-ray enlargement studies. Because less x-radiation is required, smaller focal-spot sizes may be used.

Without intensifying screens, medical radiography as we know it today would be impossible. For example, consider a screen-film exposure of the abdomen. A typical technique might be 75 kVp and 20 mAs (400 mA, 0.05 seconds). Compare this with

---

*Spectral matching occurs when the color sensitivity of film is matched to the spectrum of light produced by the intensifying screen.

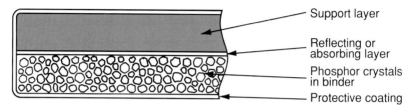

Figure 4–4 Cross Section of an Intensifying Screen.

a direct exposure technique at the same kVp, which would require 1000 mAs or more. Even if patient radiation exposure were not a consideration, most x-ray tubes could not tolerate the heat generated by exposures of this magnitude.

Screen Structure

A screen consists of a layer of tiny phosphor crystals bonded together in a suitable binder and coated in a smooth, uniform layer on a plastic, paper or cardboard support **(Figure 4–4)**. A protective coating is applied over the external surfaces of these layers to guard against abrasion, moisture and staining, and to permit cleaning. An anti-curl layer is often applied to the back of the support to help maintain flatness of the screen. In addition to the protective coating and phosphor layer, screens frequently contain a thin layer between the support and phosphor. This layer sometimes contains a light-reflecting material. In other cases it may contain a light-absorbing material.

Most commercially available screens have phosphor layers with thicknesses within the range of about 70 to 250 micrometers (μm) [250 millionths of a meter]. Phosphor crystal sizes typically fall within the range of about 3 to 15 μm, and the thickness of the protective coating ranges from about 8 to 20 μm.

FACTORS AFFECTING SCREEN EMISSION

The following summary identifies some of the factors affecting the luminance or brightness of light emitted by fluorescent intensifying screens.
1. X-ray absorption
    a. Phosphor type
    b. Amount of phosphor (thickness and packing density)
    c. Beam quality of the aerial image
    d. Single or double screen-film combination
2. Phosphor particle size
3. Light-reflecting or absorbing layers
4. Light-absorbing pigments or dyes in phosphor layer
5. Screen conversion efficiency
6. Temperature

Phosphor Type

Phosphors differ in their x-ray absorption characteristics. Two physical requirements for the chemical elements making up a highly absorbing phosphor are a reasonably high atomic number and a high physical density (mass per unit volume). The density of the phosphor is important in determining the screen thickness needed for a given amount of phosphor.

Amount of Phosphor

If other factors remain unchanged, increasing the thickness and therefore the amount of phosphor in a screen increases its x-ray absorption and light output. However, there are practical limits to screen thickness. The most important of these is the increased image blur associated with increased phosphor thickness. For a given phosphor thickness, if the phosphor is packed more densely (packing density increased), light output is also increased. This occurs without an appreciable increase in image blur. After a certain thickness is reached, much of the light generated deep in the phosphor layer is absorbed before reaching the screen surface. So there is little gain in light output with increasing thickness beyond this point.

Beam Quality of the Aerial Image

The beam quality of the aerial image is affected by the x-ray beam produced by the tube, total filtration, and anything in the beam path (for example, patient, tabletop, and grid) that influences the x-ray spectrum of the beam reaching the detector. The x-ray beam quality of the aerial image influences the amount of energy absorbed by the screen. Beam quality of the aerial image refers to the "hardness" or penetrating power of the x-ray beam incident upon the image receptor, and is affected by:
- the kVp and waveform applied to the x-ray tube (single-phase or three-phase),
- beam filtration,
- the body part being examined, which both filters the x-ray beam and generates scattered radiation,
- the use of a grid or an air gap to remove scattered radiation, and
- the filtering effect and scattering action of the examining table and cassette front through which the beam passes.

The effect of the beam quality on x-ray absorption and light output also depends on the atomic structure and the phosphor's constituent chemical elements. If other factors are held constant, the greater the x-ray energy absorbed or deposited in the screen, the greater the amount of light emitted.

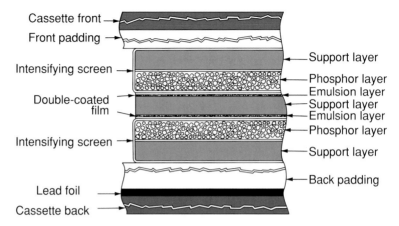

Figure 4–5   Cross Section of a Loaded Cassette. This diagram shows the screen-film configuration most commonly used in medical radiography, enclosed in a light-proof container called a cassette. A double-coated film is sandwiched between two intensifying screens and enclosed in a cassette to provide good screen-film contact and protection from light and damage. The back of many cassettes is covered on the inside with a sheet of lead foil to prevent backscattered x-radiation from reaching the screen-film combination. (Components in this diagram are not drawn to scale.)

Single or Double Screen-Film Combinations

A single screen is combined with single-coated film (emulsion on one side only) for examinations such as mammography and the extremities, where it is critical that image blur be minimized. X-ray absorption may be increased by the use of two intensifying screens, one on each side of a film coated with emulsion on both sides. This double screen-film combination is the configuration most commonly used in medical radiography (**Figure 4–5**). In the *standard* dual-screen, dual-emulsion film system, both screens are identical in thickness, as are the emulsions coated on both sides of the film. This configuration has been in common use for decades.

Some intensifying screen pairs are **asymmetric**, that is, the front screen is somewhat thinner than the back screen. This difference in thickness equalizes the x-ray absorption and light output of the two screens, producing equal film blackening effects on both sides of the x-ray film.

Consider the effect of using two screens of equal thickness (**Figure 4–5**). For simplicity, assume in this example that the x-ray beam contains photons of only a single energy (monoenergetic). If the two screens have the same thickness, they will each absorb the *same percentage* of photons from the x-ray beam. For example, if the front screen (the one closest to the x-ray tube) absorbs 20% of the incident radiation, the back screen will absorb only 16% (20% of the remaining 80% of the radiation that reaches it). Therefore, where screens are designed to have high x-ray absorption to reduce exposure, a front screen thinner than the back screen may be desirable. A further development in image receptor design incorporates the use of asymmetric screens with asymmetric film (**Figures 5–6** and **5–7**).

Phosphor Particle Size

If other factors remain unchanged, increasing the size of the phosphor crystals tends to increase the brightness of screen light emitted. From a practical standpoint, however, phosphor: layer thickness, atomic number, and packing density are the dominant parameters of screen design.

Light-Reflecting or Absorbing Layers

Introducing a reflecting or absorbing layer between the phosphor and the support can also affect screen light emission (**Figure 4–4**). When an x-ray photon is absorbed, the resulting light photons emerge from the phosphor crystal in all directions. About half of these photons travel toward the back of the screen away from the surface in contact with the film. However, if the layer between the phosphor and support contains a reflecting material, the light reaching it will be redirected back toward the screen surface that is in contact with the film. This increases the light output emerging from the screen to expose the film. Conversely, if the layer between the phosphor and support contains a light-absorbing material, the light reaching it will make no contribution to exposing the film.

Such a layer affects not only the intensity of light emission but also the image blur produced by the screen. Some screens employ a reflecting or absorbing *support* instead of a separate layer for reflection or absorption.

Light-Absorbing Pigments or Dyes in Phosphor Layer

A light-absorbing dye or pigment is incorporated in the binder of the phosphor layer of some screens. The dye preferentially absorbs light photons along a longer path, that is, those not emitted directly toward the screen, resulting in image blur. This method also reduces the amount of light emitted by the screen. Screens of this type may have a gray, pink or yellow tint, depending upon the pigment or dye that is used as an absorber (**Figure 4–6**).

Screen Conversion Efficiency

Thousands of light quanta can be generated by the interaction of a single x-ray photon with one phosphor particle. The ratio of the total light energy (number of

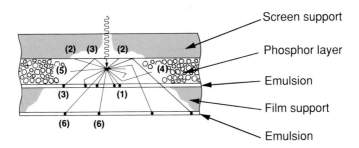

Figure 4–6 Light Photons Emitted by a Phosphor Crystal in an Intensifying Screen. **(1)** Light photons travel through the phosphor layer and are absorbed in the front emulsion layer of the film. **(2)** Some are absorbed by the screen support. **(3)** The light is reflected by the screen support and absorbed by the film. **(4)** The light is then scattered by another phosphor particle and absorbed by pigment in the phosphor layer. **(5)** Some light is absorbed by dye or pigment in the phosphor layer. **(6)** The light then travels through the front emulsion layer of the film and the film support to be absorbed in the opposite emulsion; this is known as crossover of light (see **Figure 4-9**).

photons times the energy of each photon) emitted by the screen to the x-ray energy absorbed in the screen is referred to as the **screen conversion efficiency**. The efficiency with which x-ray energy is converted to light differs among phosphor types.

Screen conversion efficiency should not be confused with *intrinsic efficiency* or *phosphor conversion efficiency*, which is the ratio of total light energy generated in the phosphor *crystal* to the x-ray energy absorbed in the screen. Not all of the light produced by the phosphor emerges from the screen. Overall screen efficiency is only about *one half* the intrinsic efficiency of its constituent phosphor material, due primarily to light loss within the screen.

Temperature

The temperature range encountered in most radiology departments does not significantly affect screen emission. However, as a matter of interest, screen emission increases as screen temperature is lowered. This effect tends to be offset by the decreasing speed of film as temperature is lowered, so the speed of the screen-film combination remains relatively constant.

SCREEN CATEGORIES

One method used to classify screens is to separate them into categories according to their relative light output or speed. Intensifying screens are

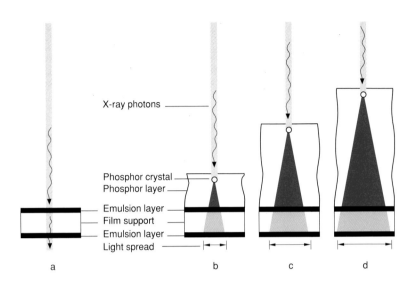

X-ray photons

Phosphor crystal
Phosphor layer

Emulsion layer
Film support
Emulsion layer
Light spread

a   b   c   d

Figure 4–7 Effect of Screen Thickness on Light Spreading. **(a)** Since direct exposure films do not use intensifying screens, there is no spreading of light from emulsion layer to emulsion layer. **(b-d)** For intensifying screens, the thicker (faster) the screen, the greater the lateral spreading of light before it reaches the film, and the greater the blurring of the image. This figure is greatly oversimplified; for in reality, light emitted by the phosphor crystals does not follow a smooth conical path to the film (see **Figure 4-6**).

available in a number of different speeds. While screens vary in speed, the factor of practical significance is **system speed** (a combination of screen speed, film speed, spectral matching between screen and film, and processing).

In photography or radiography, speed is inversely related to the radiation exposure (light or x ray, respectively) required to produce a given film blackening effect. That is to say, a fast screen (one having high speed) requires less x-ray exposure to provide a given film blackening effect. A slow screen is said to have low speed and requires more x-ray exposure. If the same exposure is used for both, a fast screen will produce a greater film blackening effect than a slow screen. Therefore, a fast screen has high light output for a given incident x-ray exposure; whereas a slow screen emits a relatively low amount of light for the same x-ray exposure.

For convenience, screens are often divided into three categories according to speed: slow (also referred to as detail or high resolution); medium (universal, midspeed, general, average or par); and fast (high speed) **(Figure 4–7)**. The relationships among screen speed categories are usually described by a comparison with one of them as a standard. Since medium-speed, calcium-tungstate screens were widely used for many years, they are often taken as a basis for comparison. The high absorption and conversion efficiency of rare-earth phosphors can be used to produce ultra-fast screens. These screens are useful in procedures such as angiography

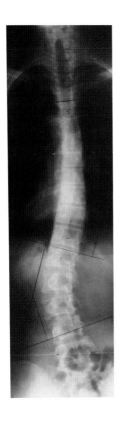

Figure 4–8 Full Vertebral Column Examination. A 1200-speed film, screen-film combination is suggested for radiography of the entire vertebral column for evaluation of scoliosis. In this illustration, a "Clear-Pb" AP/PA Wedge Filter was used with a uniform speed intensifying screen-film system (modified, courtesy of Nuclear Associates, Carle Place, NY).

and evaluation of the full vertebral column for scoliosis, where repeated examinations emphasize the importance of minimizing patient radiation exposure **(Figure 4–8)**.

By design, radiation therapy equipment produces very high radiation fluences for treatment purposes. To accommodate the need to produce localization and verification images as a part of this process, very slow image receptors must be employed.

Meaningful measurement of screen speed is complicated. Such measurements must contain information about the spectral emission (the color distribution) of the screen light, and the ratio of the light energy emitted to the x-ray energy absorbed (screen conversion efficiency) for a number of different exposure conditions. This information is necessary to permit calculation of system speeds when the screens are combined with different films and processing systems.

In practice, measurement of the response of the entire system (screen-film combination, plus processing) to x-ray exposure is more useful than the response of an individual component within a system, such as screen speed.

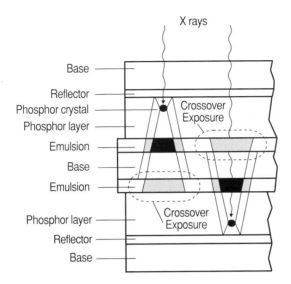

Figure 4–9 Crossover of Light. Light from an x-ray screen is given off in all directions. In this illustration, light is shown as a cone passing from an intensifying screen through the adjacent emulsion and base to the opposite emulsion. The segment of the emulsion of the film exposed adjacent to the screen is larger than the phosphor crystal. A larger area of the opposite emulsion is exposed by the crossover of light.[6]

LIGHT DIFFUSION

The preceding discussion focused on the construction and functioning of fluorescent intensifying screens, with an emphasis on factors that influence light emission or speed. The benefits derived from the use of intensifying screens have been listed. In the real world, however, no benefits exist without costs, only compromises among different factors.

As intensifying screens improve the overall speed of a screen-film image receptor, they also degrade the image by introducing a blurring of the information that exists in the aerial image. That is, an image produced using a screen-film system has increased image blur relative to that of an image obtained using film alone without screens (direct exposure). This blurring of the screen image results from the lateral spreading of light as it travels through the screen, from the phosphor crystal from which it originates, toward the film where it is recorded (**Figure 4–9**).

In general, those factors that increase the brightness (speed) of the light emitted by the screen also increase light spreading and image blur. Conversely, those factors that reduce screen speed usually decrease light diffusion and image blur. The following factors summarize the effects of screen construction on screen speed and light spreading. In each instance, it is assumed that all other factors are held constant.

1. Increasing phosphor layer thickness increases speed and light divergence (**Figure 4–9**).
2. Using a reflecting layer or support increases speed and light spread (**Figure 4–4**).
3. Using an absorbing underlayer or support decreases speed and light divergence (**Figure 4–4**).
4. Adding a light-absorbing pigment to the phosphor binder decreases speed and light divergence (**Figure 4–6**).
5. Decreasing the size of the phosphor particles decreases speed and light divergence.

There is one important exception to the generalization about the relationship between screen thickness and speed. It is possible to increase x-ray absorption and screen speed without increasing screen thickness or light divergence by using a phosphor of a higher packing density and higher atomic number. These are some of the factors that make rare-earth phosphors preferable to calcium tungstate.

Even the thinnest, slowest screens exhibit greater image blur than a film exposed directly to x rays. However, virtually all medical radiography is done with intensifying screens, showing that the advantages of screens usually more than compensate for the degradation in image quality associated with their use. Furthermore, screen blur is only one factor in overall image quality. Improved overall image quality and reduced patient radiation exposure make high-resolution, screen-film image receptors universally preferred over direct-exposure film techniques.

SCREEN CARE

Screens must be inspected and cleaned regularly to keep them free of dirt and foreign material. Such material can interfere with a proper diagnosis by casting an unwanted shadow or **artifact** that degrades the image, or by causing poor screen-film contact, resulting in increased image blur (**Figure 4–10**). An *artifact* is any appearance on a radiograph that is not representative of a structure within the patient. Grit or foreign material can also scratch or damage the screens, thereby necessitating early replacement.

To avoid the problems associated with dirt and foreign material, it is essential that high standards of housekeeping be maintained to keep darkroom and film-loading areas clean. If storage is necessary in the darkroom, it is preferable to use closed-door cupboards rather than open shelves where dust settles readily on horizontal surfaces. In general, non-essential storage in the darkroom should also be minimized. For example, cardboard boxes should not be opened inside the

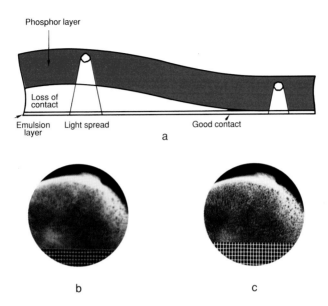

Figure 4–10 Screen-Film Contact. **(a)** The screen is separated from the film on the left of the diagram. This separation may have been caused by a pocket of trapped air, foreign material on the screen, surface irregularities arising from damage to the cassette, or improper mounting of the screens. This separation causes the light to travel farther to reach the film, spreading farther laterally than the light from the portion of the screen on the right side of the diagram, which is in close contact with the film. The increased light spreading results in increased image blur. Representative radiographs demonstrate the effect of **(b)** poor screen-film contact on image blur, compared with an image made with **(c)** good screen-film contact.

darkroom—they can generate large amounts of dust. In addition, eating, drinking, and smoking should be prohibited in the darkroom.

Screens should be cleaned according to the manufacturer's instructions to avoid damage to screen surfaces. For example, some solutions recommended for use with calcium-tungstate screens are not suitable for use with ultraviolet-emitting screens because of the residue they leave on the screens. This residue contains an *optical brightener*, which adheres to the screen surface and interferes with ultraviolet emission. The presence of such brighteners can be detected by examining the screen with a source of ultraviolet radiation, such as the BLB (black light bulb) fluorescent lamp used in duplicating printers.

Care must be taken to keep the screen surface dry and to avoid soiling and staining that may permanently damage the screen. One should also avoid touching screen surfaces. Common sources of screen artifacts include medications, such as nasal sprays, that reach the screen as a result of sneezing or

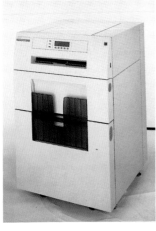
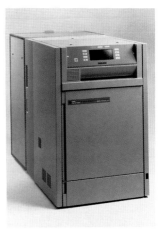

a   b

Figure 4–11   Roomlight Cassette Loaders.   **(a)** A multiloader with a built-in processor with three x-ray film magazines. **(b)** A multiloader with seven supply magazines. The exposed film can be transported to a linked processor for development.

coughing, ink and pencil marks, soot, cigarette ashes, lipstick, nail polish, and processing solution splashes.

Screen manufacturers' recommendations on cleaning products and procedures must be followed for optimal screen performance.

Static electricity can attract dust particles to the screen, blocking the screen light from exposing the film. Static electricity can also cause branch-like black artifacts. An anti-static solution applied to the screens helps reduce static. Some screen cleaning solutions also contain an anti-static compound. Since low relative humidity aggravates the problem of static electricity, use a humidifier in the film-loading area during periods of low humidity.

Keep cassettes closed when not in use. This prevents dust and dirt from accumulating on the screens. Avoid scratching the screen when loading and unloading film.

CASSETTES

The screen-film combination used to record the x-ray image must be placed in a light-proof holder to protect it during transport to and from the location where it is to be exposed. This holder, called a **cassette**, usually contains one pair of screens. A film is inserted in the cassette and removed manually for each exposure (**Figure 4–5**). Roomlight cassette loaders are available that do not require a darkroom to automatically unload and reload cassettes (**Figure 4–11**).

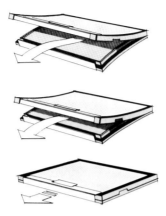

Figure 4–12 Cassette with Curved Front and Back Panels. As indicated by the arrows, air is squeezed out from between the screens and the film to maximize screen-film contact.

Exterior surfaces of the cassette should be kept clean of foreign material, such as barium or iodinated contrast media, which could cast confusing shadows on the radiograph.

A rapid serial film changer may be used for certain limited applications. These systems automatically transport exposed film away from the screens, replace it with unexposed film, and re-establish screen-film contact.

SCREEN-FILM CONTACT

Most cassettes are hinged containers made of metal or plastic. Traditionally, rigid construction and the pressure exerted by the spring latches helps keep the emulsion on each side of the film in close contact with the light-emitting surfaces of the screens. However, a problem frequently encountered with traditional cassettes is poor screen-film contact, resulting from air pockets being trapped between screens and film as the cassette is closed. These pockets sometimes arise from irregularities in the screens and cassettes or may be the result of damage and wear.

Cassettes should not be dropped or handled roughly. Dents or lack of alignment of the cover and back affect contact between the screens and film.

An improvement in cassette design, namely, the use of curved front and back panels, has greatly reduced the probability of trapping air between screens and film (**Figure 4–12**). As the cassette is closed, air is squeezed out by the rolling action of the screen surfaces coming together, thereby increasing the likelihood of good screen-film contact.

Effect of Poor Screen-Film Contact

Poor screen-film contact has a detrimental effect on the radiographic image (**Figure 4–10**). If there is a space between the screen and the film, the light from the screen must travel farther before reaching the film than in areas where the screen and the film are in close contact. The farther the light has to travel, the more it diverges or spreads laterally, tending to blur the image. Consequently, an exposure can be made in which great care has been taken to minimize image blur due to patient motion, focal-spot size, focal-film distance, and light diffusion in the screens, only to have these efforts nullified by blur resulting from poor screen-film contact.

In summary, poor screen-film contact can be caused by several factors, including:
- air trapped between screen and film,
- foreign material on the screen, and
- damaged cassettes or latches.

Testing Screen-Film Contact

The deterioration of screen-film contact in a particular cassette may be gradual and go unnoticed until it becomes severe. For this reason, a regular schedule for testing screen-film contact should be maintained. One simple test is to radiograph a wire-mesh screen placed on the cassette. The resulting test radiograph is viewed from a distance of about 2 to 3 meters. Any areas of poor contact will appear as dark regions on the radiograph. On close examination, these areas will appear blurred or fuzzy.

Detailed recommendations for testing screen-film contact are available from manufacturers of screen-film contact test tools.

Mammographic imaging requires a more stringent test for screen-film contact. Specialized test tools with fine mesh metal screens (about 40 copper wires per inch) must be used to demonstrate effects that would escape detection using the standard test tool, which is adequate for testing *general* radiographic cassettes. (**Figure 4–13**).

SUMMARY

Film is extremely sensitive to visible light, but relatively insensitive to x rays. Intensifying screens optimize x-ray absorption and convert x-ray energy into

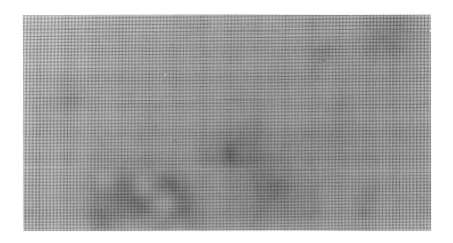

Figure 4–13 Radiograph of a Mammographic Screen-Film Contact Test Tool. Mammographic imaging has more stringent image blur requirements than conventional radiographic imaging. Radiographic details that include punctate calcifications or minute vascular patterns could be obscured by even minimal loss of screen-film contact. A specially designed mammographic test tool uses a fine metallic wire mesh screen to demonstrate areas of reduced screen-film contact. The regions of increased optical density on this test radiograph indicate areas of poor screen-film contact.

light, while maintaining spatial fidelity (faithfully reproducing the information in the aerial image).

Compared with direct-exposure film technique (non-screen), intensifying screens increase both speed and image blur. As a result of the increased speed, however, associated benefits arising for other technical factors (reduced motion blur, smaller focal-spot size) result in overall improvement in image quality. Furthermore, the use of intensifying screens reduces patient radiation exposure 10 to 100 times or more when compared with direct-exposure technique.

Due to the interdependence between intensifying screens and film, it is of limited practical value to characterize one without the other. The following chapter discusses film as the essential component in medical radiographic imaging. In the process, the interrelationship between screens and film is more thoroughly described.

Chapter 5
Recording the Image–Film

In its early form, fluoroscopy—without the aid of electronic image intensifiers and video displays—was the predominant method of x-ray imaging and diagnosis. A major disadvantage of these primitive systems was the lack of a permanent record of the fluoroscopic image. Since those early days, advances in x-ray film technology allow permanent recording of high-quality, low-dose medical radiographic images on x-ray film. This chapter investigates the technology and practical application of film in medical imaging.

X-ray film is much more sensitive to visible light than to x-radiation. The purpose of x-ray screens is to efficiently absorb x-ray energy and convert it into visible light, while faithfully maintaining the information contained in the aerial image. The cassette is the physical enclosure that maintains contact between the film and the screen in a light-tight, rigid enclosure. The cassette must neither introduce artifacts into the image, nor significantly absorb x-radiation from the aerial image.

FILM TYPES

Direct-Exposure Films

Before high-quality intensifying screens were in common use, medical radiographic imaging was performed using direct exposure of x-ray film in a cardboard light-tight holder (**Figure 5–1**). This technique was used for certain examinations, such as studies of the distal extremities where radiation risk to the patient was minimal, and where an image with reduced screen blur was desired. To improve the absorption of x rays in the aerial image, film created for use without intensifying screens was designed with thicker emulsion layers. Direct-exposure (non-screen) film absorbs three to four times more x-radiation than screen-type film when used in direct-exposure technique. Therefore, when direct-exposure technique is required, the use of direct-exposure film over screen-type film (without screens) requires significantly less patient radiation exposure. In spite of thicker emulsions, most of the incident x-radiation of the aerial image is not absorbed by the film. The radiation passes through and exits the film and therefore does not contribute to the useful image. Direct-exposure technique, however, requires 10 to 100 times or more radiation exposure than that required for screen-film technique.

Direct-exposure films are less sensitive to light than screen-type films and therefore should not be used with intensifying screens. However, since direct-exposure films are sensitive to both light and x rays, photographic and radiographic film should always be protected against stray, non-image forming radiation that can partially expose the film, causing film fog* during storage and handling.

---

*Fog is defined as film density arising from factors other than the radiation used for imaging.

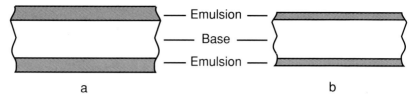

Figure 5–1 Non-Screen vs Screen Film. While the base of both radiographic films have the same thickness, **(a)** direct exposure film, such as non-screen film, is coated with considerably more silver halide emulsion than is **(b)** screen film. Non-screen film is primarily sensitive to the direct exposure of x-radiation, while screen film responds more readily to light given off by fluorescent intensifying screens.

X-ray film may be kept in its cardboard packaging for weeks or months. However, packaging boxes, which are light-tight, offer no protection from x-radiation. Film fog may be caused by small amounts of scattered x-radiation (exposures as low as 1 milliroentgen) or from naturally occurring background radiation during the time between film manufacture and the time of processing.

Screen-Type Films

X-ray film is capable of recording either the aerial x-ray image directly or the fluorescent image produced by intensifying screens (**Figure 5–1**). Specific films may be made expressly for use with specific intensifying screens. Film can also be designed to have greater sensitivity to certain colors of light. This allows the color sensitivity of the film to be matched to the spectrum of light produced by the screen (**Figure 5–2**). Most x-ray film used today is orthochromatic—it is highly sensitive to the green visible light produced by primarily green-emitting, rare-earth screens. These films absorb light more readily than they absorb the more penetrating x-radiation. Practically all exposures in medical radiography are made with screen-film combinations because of the many advantages they offer, such as increased radiographic contrast, reduced radiation exposure to the patient, and shortened exposure times, which decrease image blur from involuntary motion.

X-RAY FILM

The x-ray aerial image exiting the patient is fleeting, lasting only for the duration of the x-ray exposure, typically, a fraction of a second. Intensifying screens convert this fleeting x-ray image to a comparably brief visible light image. To produce a long-lasting image that may be studied carefully and repeatedly, the screen light image is transferred to another type of image receptor—an x-ray film. The x-ray film, processed in a manner similar to the way black and white photographs are produced, becomes the radiograph—the lasting or **archival** record of the x-ray image.

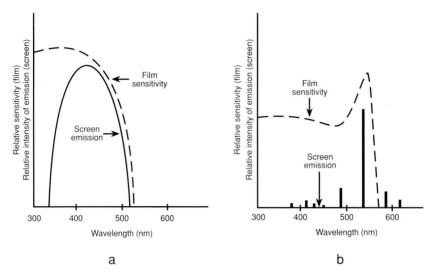

Figure 5–2 Spectral Sensitivity of Typical X-ray Film Emulsions and the Spectral Emission of Corresponding Intensifying Screens. For optimal performance, the spectral sensitivity of x-ray film must be matched to the emission characteristics of the intensifying screens used. This figure shows screen emission (solid line) and film sensitivity spectra (dashed line) for typical **(a)** blue and **(b)** green systems.

Composition of X-ray Film

X-ray film generally consists of a flexible support, or **base**, coated with a very thin adhesive *subcoating* that binds the emulsion to the base (**Figure 5–3**). The **emulsion** is a gelatin containing a silver compound. The emulsion is usually coated on both sides of the base (double-emulsion film) in a layer from 3 to 5 micrometers (μm) thick. The use of double-emulsion film with a spectrally (color) matched pair of screens decreases the radiation exposure required to produce the appropriate film blackening effect, thereby reducing radiation exposure to the patient. Dual-emulsion, dual-screen systems are said to be "faster" than single-emulsion, single-screen systems, but a compromise often comes with this increased speed—increased image blur. Examinations that require minimal image blur, such as mammography and the extremities, often use a single screen with a single-emulsion film.

Gelatin

Gelatin is used in x-ray film to keep the silver compound (in the form of silver halide microcrystals or grains) well-dispersed. Since gelatin is relatively stable it adds reasonable permanence to the emulsion before and after processing. The gelatin also permits rapid processing because it is easily penetrated by developer and fixer solutions.

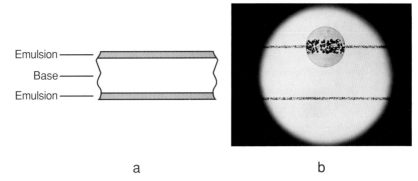

Emulsion

Base

Emulsion

a   b

Figure 5–3 Microphotograph of a Cross Section of X-ray Film. **(a)** Schematic of an x-ray film compared to **(b)** a microphotograph of a cross section of an x-ray film showing the coating of sensitive emulsion on both sides of the support. The inset in (b) shows the silver halide crystals in the emulsion.

Overcoat

Each emulsion has an overcoat of protective material to lessen the possibility of damage to the film's sensitive surface. Some protective coatings also contain compounds to improve their transport through serial film changers.

Support

The film base or support provides the appropriate degree of strength, stiffness, and flatness for handling and good dimensional stability. Film base is usually blue-tinted, with a thickness of about 180 μm. Made from a transparent plastic, the film base absorbs very little water (which is important in automatic processing) and it meets slow-burning and other safety requirements of the American National Standards Institute, Inc. (ANSI).

Silver Halide

As seen under a microscope (**Figure 5–3**), the emulsion is made up of innumerable tiny microcrystals or photographic grains of silver halide suspended in gelatin. For most medical x-ray films, these microcrystals average about 1 μm in diameter. The term **silver halide** describes a compound of silver combined with a member of the halide family of elements: bromine, chlorine or iodine. Silver bromide microcrystals containing small amounts of iodide are commonly used in x-ray film emulsions.

When the microcrystals in this sensitive emulsion absorb energy from x rays or light, a physical change takes place to form the so-called **latent image**. This image is called "latent" because it cannot be detected by ordinary physical methods. However, when exposed film is processed in a solution called a **developer**, a chemical reaction called *reduction* takes place. Reduction of the exposed

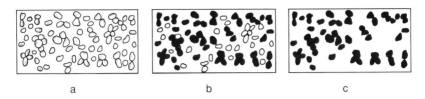

a   b   c

Figure 5–4 Processing Action in X-ray Film Emulsion. **(a)** A schematic showing the distribution of silver halide grains with the gray areas indicating the latent image produced by exposure. **(b)** During the development process, metallic silver (black) is produced in the exposed grains. **(c)** In the fixing process, the unexposed silver halide grains are removed.

microcrystals of silver compound causes tiny masses of black metallic silver to be formed, leaving the unexposed crystals essentially unaffected (**Figure 5–4**). The unexposed silver is removed from the film base as part of the fixing process.

After processing, each speck of metallic silver absorbs some of the light from the viewbox, producing the many **optical densities** or shades of gray in the image, ranging from light gray to black. Conversely, areas where the unexposed silver was removed produce clear areas on the radiograph. This allows the clear areas to appear white as the viewbox light reaches the eyes of the observer.

For many years, emulsions were made from silver halide grains that were three-dimensional and irregular in shape (**Figure 5–5a**). More recently, tabular grain emulsions have been developed. Tabular grains have a relatively larger surface area, are thinner, and are similar in shape to a guitar pick (**Figure 5–5b**).

Crossover-Control Dye

Tabular grain emulsions have a relatively high surface area that allows higher levels of optical sensitizing dyes to be absorbed by the grain (**Figure 5–6**). This high level of optical sensitizing reduces crossover by absorbing more of the light energy traveling through the emulsion. Even greater reduction in crossover can be achieved by coating a crossover control layer between each emulsion layer and the support. This layer contains an absorbing dye that reduces crossover to essentially zero. Dual-receptor, zero-crossover film, initially designed for chest imaging, has been developed for use with asymmetric screens (**Figure 5–7**).

THE LATENT IMAGE

Without the *amplification* that the latent image triggers, radiography as we know it today would not exist. It is possible to supply enough energy to the emulsion by exposure alone to convert the silver halide microcrystals *directly* to metallic silver. This process, known as photolysis or printout, produces an image without the aid of the chemical reactions used in ordinary film processing. However,

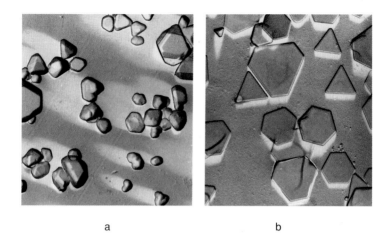

a   b

Figure 5–5 Comparison of Conventional Silver Halide Crystals with Tabular Grains. **(a)** Note the irregularly shaped silver halide crystals in conventional radiographic film, compared with **(b)** the flat tablet-like grains found in tabular grain film. Tabular grains can be dispersed more evenly throughout the emulsion. [6]

---

this method is never used in medical imaging. The radiation exposure required would be hundreds of millions of times greater than that required when a developing solution is used to convert the silver bromide into metallic silver. Obviously, such exposures are neither practical nor safe for patients or x-ray tubes. Therefore, the next section examines the formation of the latent image and its conversion to film blackening by the chemical reaction of the developer.

Formation of the Latent Image

The latent image is formed when silver halide microcrystals in film are exposed to the light emitted from intensifying screens. The following scientific model is commonly used to describe the formation of the latent image.

When a light photon from an intensifying screen is absorbed by a grain in the emulsion, its energy removes an electron from a halogen atom in the silver halide crystal. The removal of an electron is called reduction. This "free" negatively charged electron or photoelectron then drifts inside the crystal.

Eventually, the electron is caught by a "trap" or "sensitivity speck" in the crystal. Such traps can be imperfections in the crystal structure or chemicals in or on the grain that may have been introduced during the emulsion-making process. In any case, the effect is to hold the negatively charged electron at least temporarily in one place.

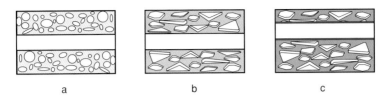

a   b   c

Figure 5–6 Crossover Control Radiographic Films. **(a)** Conventional screen-film systems utilize irregularly shaped silver halide crystals in the x-ray film. Approximately one-third to one-half of the light emitted from the fluorescent intensifying screens crosses over to the opposite emulsion. **(b)** A light-absorbing dye is used in tabular grain emulsions. This dye minimizes light spreading, reducing crossover to approximately one-half the crossover normally associated with screen-film systems, resulting in reduced image blur. **(c)** A dual-receptor, asymmetric, screen-film system uses an anti-crossover layer on the x-ray film support to completely eliminate the crossover of light. This orange dye is bleached out in the developer during processing.

Silver ions, which exist naturally in the crystals, can be thought of as atoms that are missing an electron. Positively charged silver ions tend to migrate toward the negatively charged trapped photoelectron at the sensitivity speck, which then attracts another negatively charged photoelectron. This process results in the formation of an atom of metallic silver at the trap sight. Because of its effect on the crystal structure, this new silver atom makes the trap still more effective in trapping additional photoelectrons. These additional electrons in turn attract more ions, forming more silver atoms. When this cluster becomes sufficiently large, it becomes a "development center" on the crystal.

Most chemical reactions proceed in two directions simultaneously: forward and reverse. In this case, a single atom of silver can revert back to an electron and silver ion, if it is not joined by another silver atom relatively quickly. As the number of silver atoms increases at a single trapping site, the stability of the sensitivity speck increases. This effect on the stability of the latent image helps explain *reciprocity law failure*, which will be discussed later.

DEVELOPMENT OF THE SILVER HALIDE CRYSTAL

Development of the crystal begins at the development center. The silver acts as a catalyst, spreading the development out from the development center until the whole grain becomes an irregular mass of black silver. These development centers enable the developer solution to change the silver halide crystal to metallic silver.

The ultimate effect of development is to tremendously amplify the effect of light striking the film. In normal development, only the grains that have absorbed sufficient light photons to form development centers will develop into an image.

These individual developed silver grains are too small to be seen under normal viewing conditions. What is seen is a non-uniform density distribution or

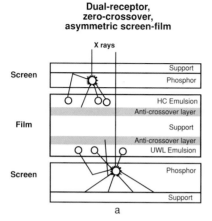

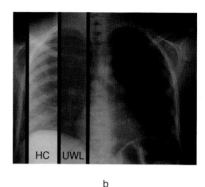

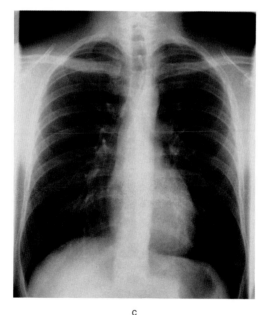

Figure 5–7   Dual-Receptor, Zero-Crossover Technology. **(a)** A dual-receptor system uses asymmetric screens (that is, thinner phosphor layer on front, thicker phosphor layer on back) with a zero-crossover asymmetric film. The film consists of a high contrast (HC) emulsion (front) and an ultra-wide latitude (UWL) emulsion (back) coated on a support having an anti-crossover layer. Conventional images on dual-emulsion film contain two essentially identical images back-to-back on the same support. With dual-crossover technology, an image on a single sheet of film can be a composite of the two separate images on each side of the support. **(b)** A chest radiograph made using zero-crossover, dual-receptor technology is shown, with strips of the front (HC) and back (UWL) emulsions removed. **(c)** A representative radiograph of the chest using dual-receptor, zero-crossover technology without compromising the lung fields.

slightly granular pattern that results from the random spatial distribution of the developed grains. This density distribution is the *graininess* with which we are familiar in amateur photography. The grainy appearance on x-ray film is the pattern seen in a film exposed uniformly to light from a source other than a screen. The much coarser pattern seen in a screen exposure is *quantum mottle*, not graininess (see Chapter 7). Larger silver halide crystals intercept more light than smaller grains. This greater efficiency in capturing light is precisely what makes faster films possible. Larger silver halide crystals by virtue of their size have higher film granularity.

Once the exposed silver halide grain has been developed, additional steps are required to make the image permanent. Details on film processing can be found in Chapter 6.

In contrast to the way film responds to exposure at the microscopic level, the next section focuses on film's large-area response as seen by the unassisted eye.

FILM RESPONSE

It is often useful to be able to predict how the film blackening effect in a radiograph will be influenced by changes in x-ray exposure and processing conditions. The study and measurement of the response of film to changes in these conditions is known as **sensitometry**. A plot of film response from light or x-ray exposure is called a **characteristic curve**, which represents a film's sensitometric characteristics. We will begin our discussion of sensitometry by defining two terms: exposure and optical density.

Exposure

The term *exposure* may be used to designate the radiographic conditions, that is, kVp, mA and time, or mAs used for a certain examination. It may also be used in the somewhat more restricted sense of the actual tube current (mA) and time (seconds), or mAs used to produce a radiograph. The term *radiation exposure* may refer specifically to the patient exposure in milliroentgens (mR). The term *exposure* may also be used to refer to the *amount* of radiation, either light or x-ray, reaching a certain area of the film; the term exposure will be used in this last sense for the remainder of this discussion. Remember, however, that film blackening may be caused by direct x-ray exposure without the use of intensifying screens, or by both x-ray and light exposure when screens are used.

Exposure, then, will be defined as the amount of x-ray or light energy reaching a particular area of the film. This energy is responsible for producing a certain *optical density* on the processed film.

Exposure may be specified in absolute units: ergs per square centimeter for light or x rays. The Roentgen (R) is a measure of the exposure in air that produces a specified amount of ionization in an ion chamber (see Appendix A). One thousand mR = one R. In most cases, **relative exposure** (ratio of absolute exposures) is more convenient and just as useful as using absolute units.

The exposure received by the film is related to the kVp, mAs, FFD, and other technical factors. Appendix A contains a brief review of the effect of changing exposure factors on x-ray images.

Optical Density

Optical density *is a quantitative measure of film blackening.* In many instances, the term optical density is simply shortened to **density**. For example, the lung fields in a chest radiograph demonstrate a greater film blackening effect and therefore have a higher (optical) density than the lighter mediastinal segment of the radiograph. It is important not to confuse this term with *physical density* or *mass density*, which is defined as mass per unit volume. For example, mediastinal structures have greater (physical) density and absorb more x-radiation than the surrounding lungs.

The image in a radiograph is built up of innumerable tiny masses of metallic silver distributed throughout the emulsion layer(s) of the film. This image is viewed by the transmitted light from an illuminator or viewbox. The relative transparency (the ability of a portion of the radiograph to transmit light from the viewbox) of the various areas in the radiograph depends upon the distribution of the developed black silver masses. The degree to which the silver attenuates (absorbs), or interferes with, the transmission of light through a small area of a radiograph is related to the *amount* of silver in that area. It is this variation in the *quantity* of transmitted light that makes up the image seen by the eye.

The heavier the deposit of black silver, the greater the absorption of light, and the darker the area appears. This film blackening is defined as optical density. Regions of lower or higher optical density refer to whether more or less light is transmitted by the radiograph. The higher the optical density, the lower the amount (fluence) of light transmitted. A device called a **densitometer** is used to measure density (**Figure 5–8**).

Measuring Density

The densitometer compares the relative amounts of light *entering* a particular area on one side of the processed film with the amount of light *emerging* from the film. The measured amount of light is defined in terms of luminance, a quantitative measure of its brightness. For a small area of film, *the ratio of the incident light to the transmitted light is called the* **opacity** *of the film.* Frequently, film has opacities with large numerical values, such as 100, 1,000 or 10,000. To simplify mathematical operations with these large numbers, logarithms are used.

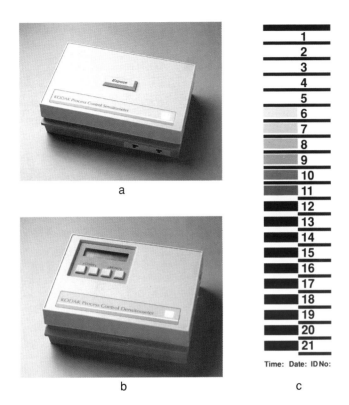

Figure 5–8 Sensitometer and Densitometer. **(a)** A process control sensitometer is shown with a **(b)** process control densitometer. **(c)** A sensitometric film strip after processing is also shown.

The common logarithm of the *opacity* is called the *optical density*. This is expressed in the form of the equation,

$$D = \log \frac{I_o}{I_t}$$

where D is density,
I_o is the original light incident on the film and,
I_t is the light transmitted by that particular area of film.

Introduction to Logarithms

A logarithm, or log, is an exponent. Logs are often used to represent and compare numbers that cover a wide range of values on the same axis of a graph, like comparing 1 and 1,000. There are three key items about logs that are important to understanding logarithmic plots, such as the characteristic curve:

1. Numbers are often expressed using exponents. When you see the word *log* think of the phrase "*the power on 10 producing...*" For example,

Number			Log
1	=	1×10^0	0
10	=	1×10^1	1
100	=	1×10^2	2

2. Because logs are exponents, **the log of the product of two numbers is equal to the sum of their logs**. That is,

Log (A x B) = Log A + Log B, just as
$10^2 \times 10^1$ = 10^3,
Log (100 x 10) = Log 100 + Log 10 = 3

3. **The log of 2 is 0.3.** This is a somewhat less intuitive concept than the others because it is not easy to visualize a fractional exponent. Nonetheless, the following is true:

Log 2 = 0.3
Log 20 = Log (10 x 2) = 1 + 0.3 = 1.3

It is often useful to know the effect of doubling the exposure to a screen-film combination. Since the horizontal axis (abscissa) of the characteristic curve is **Log Relative Exposure**, doubling the amount of exposure means adding 0.3 to the log.

For example, using **Figure 5–9**, point E1 represents a given amount of exposure and the optical density that it produces on film. To know the optical density that is produced by twice as much radiation exposure to the screen-film combination, add 0.3 to the x-axis value and find point E2. One can see the effect on optical density from doubling the exposure.

The effect of doubling the exposure again can be seen by adding another 0.3 to the x-axis value, point E3. It can be seen that the optical density did not increase as much as from E1 to E2. This is because the screen-film combination has been overexposed, that is, point E3 is beyond the straight-line portion of the characteristic curve.

Examples

Consider the measurement of optical density in these examples. When the silver in a radiograph allows 1/10 of the light to pass through, the opacity is the ratio of the original incident light to the transmitted light, that is, 10/1 or simply 10. The logarithm of 10 is 1 and, therefore, the area is said to have an optical density of 1.00. Again, if the silver allows only 1% or 1/100 of the light to pass through, the ratio is 100/1. The logarithm of 100 is 2 and, therefore, the area has an optical density of 2.00.

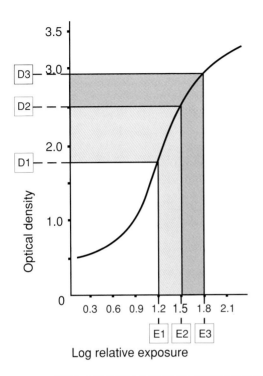

Figure 5–9 Log Relative Exposure and Optical Density. A screen-film system characteristic curve shows the output (optical density) on the y-axis resulting from input conditions (x-ray exposure) as log relative exposure on the x-axis. Doubling the input x-ray exposure is shown as an increase in log relative exposure of 0.3. Note that doubling the exposure from E1 to E2 produces a difference in optical density from D1 to D2. This density difference is greater than D2 to D3, which is produced when doubling x-ray exposure from E2 to E3.

Medical radiographs contain many different optical densities in the various areas that comprise the image. These optical densities range from about 0.30 in the relatively clear areas to more than 3.00 in the very blackest areas (**Figure 5–9**). In other words, an area of the film with an optical density of 0.30 contains enough silver deposits to allow one-half of the light produced by the viewbox to pass through the radiograph to the observer. The darkest portions of the radiograph, with an optical density of 3.00, allow only 1/1000 of the viewbox light to be transmitted.

THE CHARACTERISTIC CURVE

It is often convenient to be able to describe the characteristics of a film-process combination by relating the optical density of a radiograph to the radiation exposure required to produce that density. If a series of known exposures is given to different areas of a film and the densities produced after processing are measured, a graph can be plotted showing the density resulting from each exposure. For most applications, it is more useful to plot the relationship between density and the logarithm of relative exposure (**Figure 5–10**). In radiography, the ratios of exposures are usually more significant than the absolute values of the exposures themselves. Therefore, it is usually sufficient and more convenient to

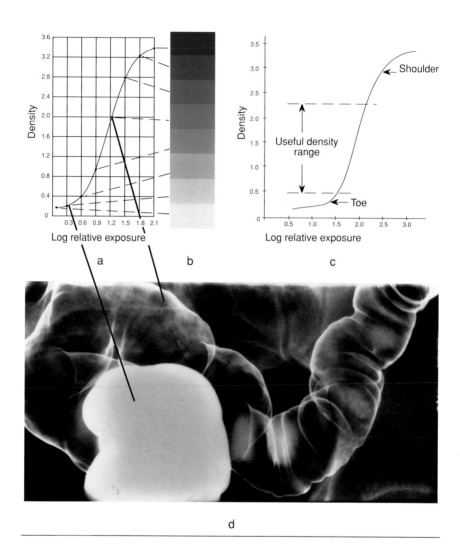

Figure 5–10 The Characteristic Curve of a Typical Medical X-ray Film. **(a)** The curve expresses the relationship between the logarithm of relative exposure (horizontal axis) and the resulting optical density (vertical axis). **(b)** In the center, a processed strip of film that was given a carefully controlled series of exposures is shown. Each step of the strip was given an exposure twice as great as that of the step below it. (a and b) Each step is connected by a dotted line to a corresponding point on the graph, which shows the density of that step and the log relative exposure that caused it. When the points corresponding to the various steps are connected, the resulting curve is called the characteristic curve, the sensitometric curve, the D log E curve or the H & D curve for the screen-film combination. **(c)** The useful density range in medical radiography is shown. **(d)** A barium-filled rectum is imaged near the toe of the curve; the aerated colon is imaged within the straight-line portion of the curve. Various shades of gray correspond to the sensitometric steps in the useful density range (c).

express the exposures to the film using a scale based on relative exposures, that is, what happens when film is exposed to twice as much x-radiation.

There are several advantages to using a logarithmic scale for the horizontal exposure axis of the characteristic curve. The most significant advantage being that exposures with a constant ratio will always be separated by the same distance on the logarithmic scale, no matter what their absolute values. Therefore, two exposures, one of which is twice the other, will always be separated by 0.3 on the logarithmic exposure scale. For example, two exposures of 2 and 4 mR would be separated by 0.3 on the log relative exposure axis.

A **sensitometer** (**Figure 5–8**) is a device that produces a series of light exposures on film with luminances having a constant ratio to one another. When the data points in **Figure 5–10** are connected by a solid line, the resulting curve is called the **characteristic curve, the sensitometric curve**, the **D log E curve** or the **H&D curve** (named after Hurter and Driffield who first used the curve with photographic films in 1890). Characteristic curves are defined for each film-process combination. Characteristic curves can be used to provide information about the relative sensitivity (speed) and contrast of a particular film or screen-film system.

Film Speed

The speed or sensitivity of a radiographic material is inversely related to the exposure required to produce a given effect. Therefore, if in **Figure 5–11**, Film A requires only one-half the exposure needed by Film B to produce a given density, Film A is said to have twice the speed or to be twice as fast as Film B. (A factor of 2 in exposure is represented by a log relative exposure difference of 0.3.) Speeds of radiographic films are often determined from the exposures required to produce a density of 1.00 above the *base plus fog* of the films (base plus fog is the optical density of the film base plus the density of the emulsion layers in areas that have not been intentionally exposed). Values of base plus fog differ owing to inherent differences in the film base used for different film types.

The speed or sensitivity of a film is indicated by the location of its characteristic curve along the log relative exposure axis. For example, in **Figure 5–11**, the curve for the faster film (A) will lie toward the left of the curve for a slower system. Therefore, compared with a slower system, a faster system requires less exposure to produce the same optical density. Conversely, the curve for a slower film (B) will lie toward the right side of the diagram in the region where the relative exposure or its logarithm is larger.

Factors Affecting Film Speed

The following factors influence the speed or exposure required to produce a given density on a film.

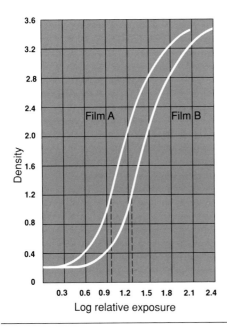

Figure 5–11 Characteristic Curves for Films Differing by a Factor of Two in Speed. Since photographic speed is inversely related to exposure, the faster or more sensitive film (A) will require less exposure than the slower film (B) to produce a density of 1.20 (a density of 1.00 and a base plus fog density of 0.20). Film A requires 10 units of relative exposure (log 10 equals 1.0), and Film B requires 20 units of relative exposure (log 20 equals 1.3) to produce the same optical density of 1.20 on each film. Note that the characteristic curves of both films have the same shape. Since their slope or steepness is the same, film contrast is also the same.

1. **Film Type** The composition of the film and the way it is manufactured affect film speed. The ingredients used in making the emulsion, the manner in which they are treated and combined, and the technique by which they are coated on the film base all play a part in determining the sensitivity of the film.

2. **Exposure Type** Significantly more exposure is required to produce a given density when the film is exposed to x rays alone than when intensifying screens are used.

In the case of screen light exposures, the sensitivity or speed of the film depends on the energy, or color, of the exposing light. The manner in which the film responds to radiation of different energies or wavelengths is called its *spectral sensitivity*. A graph that shows the relationship of the film's sensitivity to the energy or wavelength of exposing radiation is called a spectral sensitivity curve (**Figure 5–2**).

3. **Reciprocity Law Failure** The definition given for exposure implies that the response (optical density) of film to radiation of a given quality will be unchanged if technical factors (mA, time, distance, grid) are adjusted so that the mR remains constant. *The reciprocity law implies that this is the case regardless of whether long or short exposure times are used.* In other words, at a given kVp, 100 mAs would be expected to produce the same optical density on film whether the exposure was made at 1000 mA for 0.1 second or 25 mA for 4 seconds. This example of the reciprocity law is true for direct x-ray exposures, as in industrial radiography. However, when film is exposed to visible light, as from an intensifying screen, *reciprocity law failure* may occur.

For exposure times used in most medical radiography, the effect of reciprocity law failure is usually insignificant for most screen-film images. Long exposure times (in excess of one second) may produce clinically meaningful effects. In mammographic imaging, for example, exposure times requiring 2 seconds need about 15% more mAs to produce the same optical density as for exposures of under one second.

4. **Processing Conditions** Among the most important factors affecting film speed are the conditions used in processing the film after exposure. The chemical formulation of the solutions used, the way in which they are mixed and replenished, their temperatures, the manner in which they are agitated, the duration of developer and fixer immersion, and washing and drying conditions all contribute to the film's speed, contrast, and appearance.

The chemical action of the processing solutions amplifies the effect of exposure by a factor of many millions. It follows, then, that changes in processing conditions can have a significant effect on film's response. For this reason, optimal radiographic results can only be guaranteed when the film manufacturer's recommendations for screen-film combination, processing chemicals, and automatic processing conditions are followed precisely. This requires that each component of the system be made by the same manufacturer. In addition, processing conditions should be monitored systematically as part of a complete quality assurance program.

5. **Ambient Conditions** Film sensitivity may also be affected by such factors as temperature, humidity, age, chemical fumes, and storage conditions. Temperature extremes, high humidity, and atmospheres containing chemical contaminants should be avoided. Protection must also be provided from light leaks, excessive safelight exposure, x-radiation, and gamma radiation to avoid fogging film.

Fog

Fog is defined as film density arising from factors other than the radiation used for imaging. The term **base plus fog** refers to the optical density of the film base plus the density of the emulsion layers in areas that have not been intentionally exposed. The unwanted emulsion density can result from a number of factors, such as exposure of the film to heat, high humidity, chemical fumes, cosmic rays, background radioactivity in the environment, and improper or damaged safelights, as well as from less than optimal processing conditions. Part of the fog in a radiograph, even when processed as recommended, arises from silver halide crystals converted to metallic silver by the developer, in spite of the fact that they received no exposure to light or x-radiation.

Some modern films use emulsions that are coated on base material with different optical densities. These films have inherently higher base plus fog densities, which is not due to film exposure to light or x-radiation or to suboptimal processing.

If storage, handling, and processing conditions are not carefully controlled, a high fog density may be produced that adversely affects the contrast of the radiographic image.

Natural Background Radiation

Natural background radiation can, over time, fog film. Even if film is protected from man-made sources of radiation (for example, that produced by x-ray machines and radioactive materials used in nuclear medicine), it is being constantly exposed to natural background radiation. This source of film fog is sometimes confused with chemical fog and mistakenly attributed to chemical changes in the emulsion as it ages.

Natural background radiation consists of high-energy cosmic rays from outer space that penetrate the earth's atmosphere, and emissions from naturally occurring radioactive materials in our environment. Natural background radiation levels are typically low, but may accumulate over time to a level that will produce noticeable film fog. In some instances, this natural background radiation exposure may be responsible for a major portion of fog arising during storage of x-ray film. Since it is difficult to control natural background radiation, the best protection is to rotate film stock so that the oldest film is used first.

Post-Exposure to Safelight

After a radiographic film has been exposed to light, it is more sensitive to subsequent exposures to light, such as from safelights or a minimal light leak, than is unexposed film. For this reason, there will be a greater increase in film density from excessive safelight exposure if it occurs *after* normal patient exposure. The color of light transmitted by safelight filters is selected to provide only wavelengths for which the film has minimal sensitivity. Periodic testing for unwanted sources of light in the darkroom is an essential component of quality control.

CONTRAST

As in the case of exposure, the word *contrast* can take on a number of different meanings (not to be confused with contrast media such as barium). To avoid confusion, the contrast-associated terms used in this text are defined below.

Radiographic Contrast

Radiographic contrast is the term used to describe the density difference between two areas in a radiograph. When this density difference is large, the radiographic contrast is high (short-scale contrast). When the density difference is small, the radiographic contrast is low (long-scale contrast). An image with high radiographic contrast is one in which regions on the film corresponding to areas of high x-ray absorption in the patient appear very white (film is clear), while regions corresponding to areas of low x-ray absorption are very dark (film is black). In many cases, higher radiographic contrast improves the ability to differentiate structures in a radiograph. Radiographic contrast results from two distinct factors: *subject contrast* and *film contrast.*

Subject Contrast

Subject contrast is the ratio of x-ray fluences emerging from two adjacent regions of the subject. Subject contrast is a function of the pattern of x-ray fluences in the aerial image that expose the image receptor. Subject contrast depends upon factors that affect x-ray absorption in the subject (radiation quality and the nature of the subject) and upon scattered radiation.

Film Contrast

Film contrast is the component of radiographic contrast that determines how differences in x-ray fluence will be converted into differences in optical density on a radiograph. Film contrast is affected by film type, processing conditions, density level in the radiograph, fog level of the film, and type of exposure (whether screen light or direct x ray). These factors will be discussed in more detail later.

Measuring Film Contrast

The slope or steepness of the characteristic curve is related to film contrast. Consider the curves in **Figure 5–12**. Assume that both filmstrips were exposed together and processed together so that the differences between them are attributable to differences in film type. Superimposed on the curves are steps to show how density differences between steps change with exposure.

Notice how much steeper the slope is in the middle of the curve for Film B relative to the corresponding slope for Film A. Film B has a steeper slope because it produces a larger density difference for a given change in exposure than does Film A. Film B also has higher contrast than Film A. Therefore, the film with a characteristic curve that rises more rapidly, that is, a steeper curve, has higher contrast than a film with a characteristic curve that has a more gradual slope. Note that in the previous comparison of characteristic curves and film speed (**Figure 5–11**), Films A and B have the same contrast even though their speeds are different.

There are several ways of measuring the steepness (film contrast) of the characteristic curve, including *average gradient* and *contrast index.*

The **average gradient** is the slope of the characteristic curve, measured by connecting the two points on the characteristic curve that have optical densities equal to 2.00 and 0.25 above the base plus fog density (**Figure 5–13**).

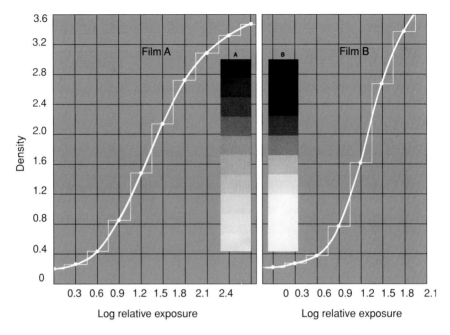

Figure 5–12 Film Contrast Differences. Radiographic contrast is the difference in optical density between two areas in a radiograph. Radiographs of a stepped-wedge taken under identical exposure conditions with two screen-film combinations A and B, and their associated characteristic curves are shown above. Film contrast is related to the slope or steepness of the characteristic curves. The density differences between steps in the middle density range of curve B are larger than those for curve A. The slope of characteristic curve B is higher or steeper than the slope of curve A. Since exposure conditions are the same for both strips, the higher radiographic contrast of B results from higher film contrast. This difference may be attributable to differences in the composition of the two films, or if the film is the same, to differences in processing conditions. Note that film contrast depends on the density level. Density differences between steps are smaller in the low-density region at the bottom (toe) and the high-density region at the top (shoulder) of the characteristic curve than they are in the middle-density region. Contrast is lower in the toe and shoulder than in the middle of the curve.

The exposure range over which the steps are well-differentiated is an indicator of film latitude. The low contrast characteristic curve A produces easily distinguishable steps over a wider range of exposures on the log relative exposure axis than does curve B.

Contrast index is the term used in processor quality control to monitor the consistency of the slope of the characteristic curve.

For light exposures in general, optical density is *not* proportional to exposure. That is to say, doubling the screen light exposure, for example, usually does not double the film density produced. It is this lack of proportionality or linearity between density and exposure that makes the characteristic curve useful in predicting density differences resulting from screen light exposure changes.

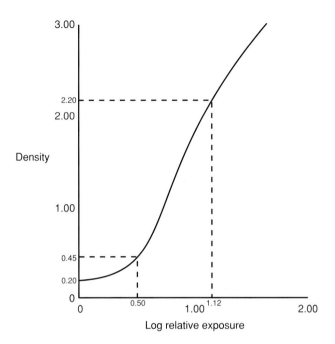

Figure 5–13 Average Gradient. The density range of 0.25 to 2.00 above the base plus fog density is used to determine the average gradient.[7]

FILM CONTRAST ILLUSTRATED

Because film can "amplify" subject contrast, many small differences in x-ray absorption within the subject can be seen.

It must be stressed that the property of film contrast is as important as speed. In medical radiography, screen-film combinations are chosen to provide images with higher radiographic contrast than the subject contrast of the aerial image.

The effect of high versus low contrast film used with intensifying screens is demonstrated in **Figure 5–14**. Frequently, the slope of the characteristic curve (average gradient) for x-ray films is 3.00 or higher in the middle-density regions.

FACTORS AFFECTING FILM CONTRAST

Contrast is one of the characteristics describing the film's response to exposure, as is speed. Furthermore, many of the elements influencing contrast are the same as those governing speed. The following factors affect contrast.

1. **Film Type** As in the case of speed, the ingredients used in film and how they are treated in the manufacturing process affect film contrast. To meet the needs of

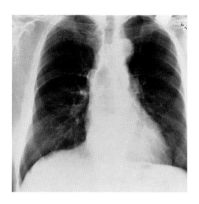 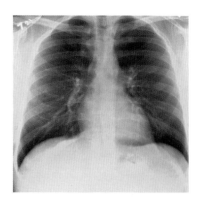

a   b

Figure 5–14 High vs Low Contrast X-ray Film in Chest Radiography. Both images were made using 110 kVp and a 12:1 ratio grid. **(a)** Note the extreme blacks and whites (short-scale contrast) in this high contrast film radiograph. Little or no detail is seen in the mediastinal area. **(b)** This radiograph used a latitude film and shows many shades of gray (long-scale contrast). Note the radiographic information in the mediastinum, the vertebral column and vascular markings.

different examinations and to suit individual preferences, manufacturers provide films with different levels of contrast.

2. **Processing Conditions** Contrast can be modified by processing conditions. The observations made concerning the effect of processing conditions on speed apply equally to contrast. It is important to follow the film manufacturer's recommendations. One should use properly mixed, fresh solutions to avoid the undesirable effects produced by solutions that have been stored too long or stored under adverse conditions. Furthermore, those responsible for processing should exercise care to avoid contamination of the processing solutions during mixing and storage. Small quantities of contaminants can significantly affect the image quality of the processed radiograph.

Chemical agents, such as accelerators, hardeners, preservatives, developing agents, and clearing agents are required to ensure the proper actions of the various processing solutions. Each of these agents may be compounded from a variety of chemicals that may differ with each manufacturer. The chemical formulation of the processing solutions—the ingredients and their relative proportions—affect the sensitometric characteristics and therefore the radiographic appearance of the films.

3. **Optical Density** Film contrast changes with density (**Figure 5–13**). Note that in the part of the curve between densities of about 1.00 and 2.00, the gradient (contrast) is higher than in regions of greater or lesser density.

Exposure conditions should be selected so that the structures of diagnostic interest in the radiograph will appear in the range of optical densities where contrast is highest. If the radiograph is *underexposed*, these structures will fall on the bottom or toe of the characteristic curve (**Figure 5–13**). If the radiograph is *overexposed*, the structures of interest will fall within the shoulder of the curve (**Figure 5–13**) corresponding to the higher optical densities. In either case, radiographic contrast will be lower, making it more difficult (or perhaps impossible) to distinguish these structures than if the structures of interest had been exposed to fall in the middle-density region.

4. **Fog** It is important to keep the fog level of film as low as possible because the radiographic effect of fog reduces film contrast. Fog density that is added to the normal fog level of a film, whether it arises from unwanted exposure, undesirable ambient conditions or improper processing, increases density the most in the lower part of the characteristic curve. This is illustrated in **Figure 5–15**, which shows the effect of excessive safelight exposure. The safelight exposure produced a "pulled-out" toe on the characteristic curve, showing a lower slope and reduced film contrast.

Latitude

Latitude describes the range of structures in the subject that can be satisfactorily imaged. Latitude can be subdivided into two categories: **exposure latitude**, which is associated with subject contrast, and **film latitude**, which is associated with film contrast. Film contrast and film latitude are reciprocally related. In other words, as film contrast increases, film latitude decreases, and vice versa.

Exposure Latitude

Figure 5–16 illustrates the effect of kVp on subject contrast. Three strips of film were exposed under an aluminum stepped-wedge at 40, 70, and 100 kVp. The strips were cut from the same sheet of x-ray film before exposure and processed together, so the differences in appearance among them are due to differences in subject contrast. Because the penetrating power of the x-radiation changes as kVp changes, the ratio of transmitted x-ray fluences, or subject contrast, between steps 7 and 12 of the aluminum wedge is greater for the 40 kVp exposure than for the 100 kVp exposure.

If it is essential that both steps 7 and 12 be imaged on a single strip, one can see that there is little latitude or margin for error in the 40 kVp exposure. If the strip had been somewhat overexposed so that the density of step 14 extended down to step 12, step 12 would then be indistinguishable from the steps on either side of it. On the other hand, if the 40 kVp strip had been underexposed so that the lower density of step 5 shifted to step 7, then step 7 would be indistinguishable from the steps on either side of it.

Next, consider steps 7 and 12 on the 100 kVp strip. Here, subject contrast is

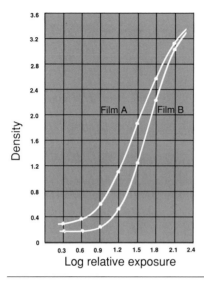

Figure 5–15 The Effect of Fog on Radiographic Film. The characteristic curve of a typical medical x-ray film is represented by A. Characteristic curve B represents an x-ray film with added fog density caused by excessive safelight exposure. This exposure "pulls out" the toe of the curve, resulting in the lower slope and reduced film contrast seen in B.

lower than for the 40 kVp strip and exposure latitude is greater. That is to say, the densities of steps 7 and 12 could be shifted several steps in either direction by a change in exposure, and the images of these steps would still be distinct from the adjacent steps. Therefore, the lower subject contrast of the 100 kVp exposure produces greater exposure latitude (long-scale contrast) than the 40 kVp exposure. On the other hand, the differences between steps are more readily apparent in the higher contrast 40 kVp exposure (short-scale contrast).

Film Latitude

Consider the characteristic curves of two films with the same speed screens, as shown in **Figure 5–12**. Film A is a wide-latitude film; Film B is a high-contrast film. The characteristic curve of Film B is steeper than Film A, owing to the higher contrast of Film B. Latitude is the range on the log relative exposure axis within which a satisfactory radiograph is produced. From this perspective, Film A has a wider latitude than Film B. As one can see from these curves, as film contrast increases, film latitude decreases.

Wide-latitude film is advantageous in radiography of the chest, where the inherent subject contrast in the aerial image is high. The use of latitude film prevents the lung fields from appearing completely black, which would obscure subtle vascular markings. Similarly, latitude film demonstrates small differences in x-ray absorption within the denser mediastinal region (**Figure 5–7**).

High-contrast film is used to visualize both osseous structures and body parts enhanced by the use of iodinated contrast media or barium (**Figures 2–9 and 2–10**). Therefore, different procedures require different types of film (latitude or contrast) to achieve specific imaging objectives. Without the proper clinical

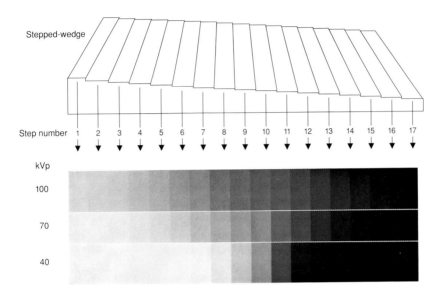

Figure 5–16 Latitude vs Contrast. Latitude is related to the range of structures in a subject that can be imaged satisfactorily. In the strip labeled 100 kVp, more steps can be seen than in the strip labeled 40 kVp. Therefore, strip 100 has greater latitude than strip 40. Strip 100 also has lower radiographic contrast than strip 40. As contrast decreases, latitude increases, and vice versa. The difference in radiographic contrast between strip 40 and 100 could be the result of either a difference in subject contrast or a difference in film contrast.

context, it is meaningless to suggest that one film is better than the other.

SUMMARY

This chapter examines some ways of measuring and describing the response of radiographic materials to exposure. It must be emphasized again that it is meaningless to treat the three components of the screen-film-process combination as separate entities. For example, one cannot specify film speed without also specifying film type, how the film was exposed, type of intensifying screen, and how it was processed.

To illustrate, consider the following. A pair of rare-earth screens that emit a high percentage of green light may require twice as much x-ray exposure to produce a given density on a blue-sensitive film as on an orthochromatic (green sensitive) film for the same processing conditions.

Furthermore, for the same screens and film, speed and contrast can change significantly, depending on the temperature of the processing solutions.

A Brief History of Screen-Film Imaging

Wet Plate vs Dry Plate Technology

The discovery of x rays in 1895 and their use in medical radiography occurred at a time when there was tremendous interest in photography, although photography was not yet an activity for the general public. In these early years, emulsions had to be kept "wet" during both exposure and development. It wasn't until the early 1870's, when silver salt and gelatin were combined to produce a dry plate, that photography became popular.

Most photographic products were emulsions coated on glass plates (**Figure 4–2**), although some papers were used as a support. In 1918, dual-emulsion film for use with a pair of intensifying screens was introduced.

The "New Photography"

Radiography was instantly dubbed the "new photography" and the so-called dry plates came into popular use. Unfortunately, up to one or more hours of x-ray exposure were needed for dense body parts, with the tube placed directly on the chest, skull or abdomen.

While the interest in intensifying screens occurred as early as January of 1896, the use of intensifying screens for radiography was not readily accepted. From early January of 1896 to March of that year, Thomas Edison tested more than 8,000 materials in his attempt to build a new incandescent lamp. He found that calcium tungstate, when used in a fluoroscopic screen, was up to six times faster than barium platinocyanide. He thought that a fluoroscopic screen should be used for "real time" imaging, and he preferred fluoroscopic "screening" to films (dry plates).

Early Screen-Film Technology

Within three months of the discovery of x rays, the first radiograph was made at Columbia University using an intensifying screen and a single-emulsion photographic plate (**Figure 5–17**). Experiments were soon underway with double-emulsion film using two intensifying screens. The radiographic image offered the advantage of a permanent record, which was not possible with

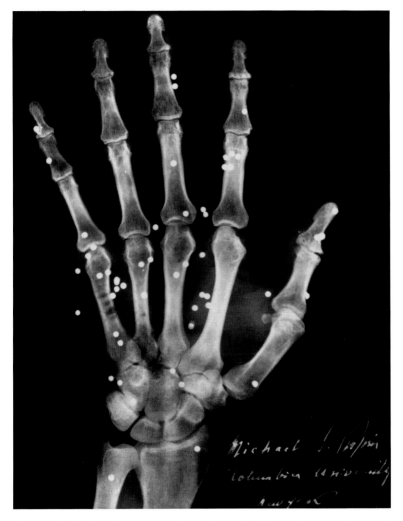

Figure 5–17 The first screen-film radiograph. This radiograph of a hand containing buckshot was made by Pupin in 1896, using an intensifying screen.[5]

fluoroscopic screening. At that time, hard copy was not important from a medical or legal standpoint; but it has become a critical issue. Unfortunately, the new intensifying screens exhibited considerable "afterglow."

For many years, glass plates were thought to be superior to film, even though glass plate images had low optical density, poor contrast, and were extremely slow. An attempt was made to use thicker emulsions on the glass plates for x-ray imaging than that usually required for photography. Glass plates, redesigned with emulsions more sensitive to x rays, continued to be popular until the mid 1920's.

Modern Screen-Film Technology

Most of the glass used for glass plates came from Belgium. The shortage of glass during World War I and the need for x-ray imaging at military installations resulted in the introduction of cellulose nitrate as a base for photographic film. Major improvements occurred with the development of a synthetic calcium tungstate compound, which ushered in the era of modern screen-film technology. A dual-emulsion film for use with a pair of calcium tungstate screens soon followed. This higher speed screen-film combination made it possible to use the Potter-Bucky diaphragm for thicker body parts. In the mid-1920's, screen-film imaging overtook glass plates, although many physicians were reluctant to give up the radiographs created with a single-emulsion direct exposure system. In the early 1920's, a cellulose acetate safety base was developed. A blue-base tint was added in the early 1930's. In the mid-1930's, non-screen film (direct exposure) extremity techniques became popular, producing high-resolution radiographs similar to glass plates at significantly lower patient radiation exposure. During World War II, some paper films were substituted for conventional x-ray films needed at military installations.

In the 1960's, a plastic base was developed that permitted a thinner based film, which minimized the parallax effect. In 1971, curved-paneled cassettes were introduced, which significantly improved screen-film contact (**Figure 4-12**). As part of this screen-film system, intensifying screens were developed using ultraviolet-emitting barium sulfate phosphors, which reduced crossover in the radiographic image. A 90-second automatic film processing (RP) system was developed in 1971. In 1991, 45-second film processing systems were introduced.

Rare-Earth Technology

In the early 1970's, medical imaging benefited from significant improvements in screen design using rare-earth phosphors. These screens utilized gadolinium oxysulfide phosphors to improve x-ray absorption and screen conversion efficiency. Orthochromatic films were developed to be primarily sensitive to the green light given off by the new rare-earth screens. Since all previous radiographic films were either blue sensitive or ultraviolet sensitive, new safelights were developed that would not fog the new orthochromatic emulsions. Rare-earth technology was used in the manufacture of extremely thin screens for significantly reduced screen blur in extremity and mammographic systems. Extremely sharp images were produced using a single screen and single-emulsion film with an anti-halation backing. Single-emulsion films eliminated crossover of light since no second emulsion existed for the light to crossover and expose.

Tabular Grain Technology

By the mid-1970's, a new film technology known as tabular grain technology was introduced. This type of film used flat, tabular silver halide crystals, placed in the emulsion parallel to the intensifying screen (**Figure 5–5**). This increased the surface area available to absorb light energy.

Dual-Receptor, Zero-Crossover Technology

In the early 1990's, newer technologies were developed to include zero-crossover systems that completely isolate one emulsion from the other. This dual-receptor technology produces a composite of two different screen-film images on a single sheet of film. A flexible, plastic film base is coated with a dye, which stops light crossover from exposing the other emulsion. This allows different clinically targeted emulsions to be coated on the front and back surfaces of the same film base. For example, a slow emulsion may be coated on the front, a fast emulsion on the back, or any combination that may be of value for specific imaging requirements.

An example of this technology was introduced in 1991. It uses dual-receptor, zero-crossover technology with a 1:6 ratio in speed between the front and back screen-film systems. The slower front screen-film combination primarily demonstrates the high contrast, sharp vascular patterns required to evaluate the lungs. Even though a lower x-ray fluence exits the denser regions of tissue, the faster posterior screen-film combination produces a darker image. This enables the viewer to evaluate the denser mediastinal structures without compromising (overexposing) the aerated lung fields (**Figure 5–7**).

Chapter 6

Automatic Film Processing and Quality Control

PROCESSING RADIOGRAPHIC FILM

Principles of Processing

Once the latent image has been formed, film must be processed to produce a visible image. No matter how carefully the patient has been positioned and technical factors have been selected to produce an optimal latent image, poor processing will always produce poor radiographs. Therefore, it is important to understand some fundamentals regarding this important step in the imaging chain.

This section focuses on automatic processing of radiographic film. Appendix E describes manual processing.

Film processing is a relatively complex series of chemical reactions, many of which occur simultaneously (**Figure 6–1**). An automatic film processor transports exposed film through a series of four sections in the machine. In each of these sections, a particular set of conditions combines to perform the following four functions.

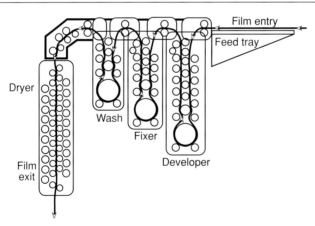

Figure 6–1 Automatic Processor with Roller Transport System. A diagram showing how the rollers transport film through the various sections of an automatic processor. The arrangement and number of components may differ from model to model but the basic processor design is the same. Typically, film is manually inserted into the processor transport system from the feed tray. The film is transported through the developer rack, the fixer rack, the wash rack, the dryer section, and exits dry and ready to interpret. The serpentine film path enables proper emulsion agitation as well as maximum chemical-to-emulsion coupling, which produces the optimum development for speed and contrast. Developer makes the latent image visible. Fixer essentially stops development, removes the undeveloped silver halide, and makes the resulting image "permanent" for keeping purposes. Washing removes chemicals to ensure proper, uniform drying and long-term archival keeping of the radiograph.

- Development: Converts the invisible latent image into a visible image composed of minute clusters of metallic silver.
- Fixing: Removes undeveloped silver halide from the emulsion and prepares the film for the remaining steps in the processing cycle.
- Washing: Removes excess chemicals from the processed film.
- Drying: Prepares the film for viewing and storage.

Film Transport

The transport system moves the film through the developer, fixer, and washing and drying sections of the processor. Optimum processing demands that each film spends exactly specified amounts of time in each section of the processor. Film moves through the processor by a system of rollers driven by a constant-speed motor. This motion also produces the required amount of chemical agitation at the film surfaces, which improves uniformity of processing.

Some modern processors are available that function at several different speeds, according to the specifications of the manufacturer. For each speed, the time of transport is carefully coordinated with temperature and chemical concentrations to achieve the desired processing results and film characteristics **(Figures 6-2a and 6-2b)**.

Water System

The water system has two functions: to wash the film and to help stabilize the temperature of the processing solutions. Some processors operate using both hot and cold water; the temperature is controlled by a mixing valve. Other processors require only a cold water supply and control the temperature with internal heating elements. Supply water must be clean and free of contaminants, sludge, and other deposits that can interfere with optimum processing.

Replenishment Systems

Film processing consumes some of the chemical components. Therefore, accurate replenishment of developer and fixing solutions is necessary to maintain consistent, high-quality film processing. The amount of replenishment required depends on the amount of film processed. Replenishment rates are determined by either total surface area or total length of film processed. Both over- and underreplenishment can lead to suboptimal radiographs.

Developing

The developer changes the latent image on film to a visible image composed of minute clusters of silver. The basic ingredients of a developer are the solvent, developing agents, accelerators or activators, preservatives, restrainers or anti-foggants, and hardeners.

1. Solvents: Water is the solvent in developer. Water dissolves and ionizes the developer chemicals. Film emulsion also absorbs water, causing it to swell; this allows the dissolved developing agents to penetrate the emulsion and to reach all silver halide crystals.

2. Developing Agents: A developing agent is a chemical compound capable of converting exposed grains of silver halide into metallic silver. The most common developing agents are hydroquinone and Phenidone.

3. Accelerators: Accelerators or activators increase the rate of chemical reaction, converting exposed silver halide grains into metallic silver (developing) at a more rapid rate. Accelerators, such as sodium or potassium carbonate and sodium or potassium hydroxide, are chemical **bases**. Bases have high pH values compared with acids, which have low pH values. The rate of chemical reaction is influenced by the pH and therefore the amount of accelerator in the solution.

4. Preservatives: An anti-oxidant preservative, usually sodium or potassium sulfite, retards the oxidation of the high pH developer solution. Preservatives also help maintain the rate of development and prevent staining of the film emulsion layer.

5. Restrainers: Restrainers protect unexposed silver halide grains from the action of the developer, minimizing film fog. Potassium bromide and potassium iodide are often used as restrainers or anti-foggants. Sometimes additional chemicals supplement the bromide ions in this function.

6. Hardeners: Hardeners prevent excessive swelling of the gelatin and damage to the film as it passes through the rollers. They act in the high-temperature, high pH developer solution.

The above summary and definitions briefly describe critical active ingredients to which additional chemical components may be added to improve stability and performance.

Some chemical ingredients are consumed during the developing process. A replenisher pump transfers fresh chemicals from an external storage container into the developer tank of the processor to restore the developer to its approximate original strength and volume. Replenishment also restores the high pH of the developer solution.

After completing the development cycle, a considerable amount of developer is retained in the gelatin of the film. Cross-over rollers remove excess developer from the film by their "squeegee" action. This prevents the high pH developer from diminishing the effect of the fixer.

Fixing

Film leaving the developer via the cross-over rollers contains metallic silver grains at the sites where x-ray photons of the aerial image exposed the film. With the exception of a small amount of chemical fog, unexposed silver halide crystals are unaffected by the developer. To complete processing, x-ray film

Kodak X-Omat processors[1]	M35/M35A[2] M35A-M	M7/M7A M7B[3] 2 minute	M6A-N/M6AW M6B[3]	M8[3]	270RA[3]	480RA[3]
Standard processing cycle (seconds)	157	127	93	93	115	93
Kwik/RA cycle (seconds)	—	—	—	—	63	45
Time in developer (seconds)	32	27	24	21.5	26 / 14.4	24 (standard) / 11.5 (Kwik/RA)
Developer °F (°C) temperature	92(33.5)	94(34.4)	95(35)	96(35.6)	94 (34.4) (standard) / 96 (35.6) (Kwik/RA)	95 (35) (standard) / 98 (36.5) (Kwik/RA)

[1]Recommended for use with Kodak RP X-Omat chemicals.
[2]Based on 43 cm of film travel, leading edge entering the processor to the trailing edge exiting the processor.
[3]Based on 35 cm of film travel, leading edge entering the processor to the trailing edge exiting the processor.

Figure 6–2a Film Processing Recommendations for KODAK Medical X-ray Films Using Standard Processing.[7]*

*Excluding mammographic films; see 6–2b.

Kodak X-Omat processors[1]		M35 M35A M35A-M M20	M6B M6-N M6A-N M6AW	M7 M7A M7B	M8	270RA[2]	480 RA[3]
Kodak film/processing cycle							
Min-R E film, extended cycle processing	Proc. Time (sec)[4]	207	172	192	NA	201	170
	Dev. Time (sec)[5]	47	47	43		53.2	46.2
	°F	95°	95°	96°		94°	95°
	°C	35°	35°	35.6°		34.4°	35°
Min-R H, Min-R M, or Min-R T films standard processing	Proc. Time (sec)[4]	140	90	122[6]	90	100	88
	Dev. Time (sec)[5]	32	24	27	21.5	26.6	23.8
	°F	92°	95°	94°	96°	94°	95°
	°C	33.5°	35°	34.4°	35.6°	34.4°	35°

[1]Kodak RP X-Omat chemicals recommended.
[2]The listed processing times are associated with a front film exit. Top film exit processing times are 214 seconds for extended-cycle processing and 107 seconds for standard-cycle processing.
[3]Some variation may occur in the listed times due to adjustable turnarounds.
[4]Processing time is based on 24 cm of film travel, leading edge entering the processor to trailing edge exiting the processor.
[5]Developer time is based on the leading edge of the film into the developer to the leading edge of the film into the fixer.
[6]Some M7 and M7A processors may have a longer standard processing time (140 seconds instead of 122 seconds). In this case, the temperature recommendation for all Kodak mammography films, standard processing, is 92°F (33.5°C).

Figure 6–2b Processing Recommendations for KODAK Min-R Films Used in Mammography (standard and extended processing cycles).[8]

must be cleared of undeveloped crystals before washing to prevent discoloration of the film with age or exposure to visible light. The gelatin coatings must also be hardened so that the film will resist abrasion and may be dried with warm air. The basic ingredients of fixer solution are:

1. Solvent: The solvent (water) diffuses into the emulsion, carrying with it the other dissolved chemicals of the fixer.

2. Fixing Agent: The fixing agent dissolves and removes the undeveloped silver halide grains from the emulsion. This action changes the unexposed areas of the film from a milky-white to a transparent appearance. The two most commonly used fixing agents (also known as **hypo**) are sodium thiosulfate and ammonium thiosulfate. If a film is improperly fixed, the remaining unexposed silver halide crystals continue to darken upon exposure to visible light after processing has been completed.

3. Preservative: Usually sodium sulfite is used as a preservative to prevent decomposition of the fixer.

4. Hardener: The hardener is usually an aluminum salt that prevents the gelatin of the emulsion from swelling excessively. It also prevents softening by the wash water or by warm air drying. Hardner also shortens drying time.

5. Acidifier: Acetic acid or other acidic compounds are used to accelerate the action of other chemicals and to neutralize any developer (high pH) that may be carried over from the developer tank.

6. Buffer: Buffers are chemical compounds that maintain a constant pH of the solution during the fixing process. When high pH developer neutralizes the low pH acidic solutions of the fixer, buffers act to maintain the pH at the desired level for optimum fixing action.

Because some chemical ingredients are consumed during the fixing process, a replenisher pump transfers fresh chemicals from an external storage container into the fixer tank of the processor. This restores the fixer to its approximate original strength and volume.

Washing

Washing removes the last traces of processing chemicals and prevents fading or discoloration. One of the important characteristics of a finished radiograph is its archival (long-term) storage capability.

Drying

A blower supplies heated air to the dryer section of the film processor. Most of the warm air is recirculated; the rest is vented to prevent buildup of excessive humidity in the dryer. The dryer temperature should be set as low as possible while still being consistent with good drying. The dryer temperature should never exceed the film manufacturer's recommendations.

Preparation of Solutions

Processing solutions are usually reconstituted from powders by the addition of water, or produced by dilution of concentrated liquid chemicals. Many facilities choose to subscribe to chemical and processor maintenance contracts. Whichever way they are produced, processor chemicals must be mixed and handled according to the manufacturer's published instructions. This includes careful control of cleanliness of receptacles, contamination, temperature, and the volume of chemicals and water used.

Environmental Considerations

The by-products of automatic film processors are waste liquid and gases. Safe and effective operation of the processor requires adequate ventilation and drainage. The user must comply with all local, state, and federal regulations regarding the introduction of waste material into the environment.

Effluent liquid from the processor contains metallic silver that is removed during fixation. Effective silver recovery minimizes the introduction of silver into the environment. A variety of methods and products are available for silver recovery. Reclaimed silver is sold as a source of revenue.

Optimum Processing Concepts

Optimum processing means:
- achieving the desired sensitometric characteristics (speed, contrast, and fog levels) in the processed image,
- presenting an artifact-free radiograph within the range of optical densities required for observer interpretation,
- producing radiographs that make the most efficient use of the x-radiation in the aerial image, thereby minimizing the radiation exposure to the patient, and
- day-to-day consistency in the sensitometric results of processing.

In order to achieve optimum processing, the film manufacturer's recommendations must be followed for:
- processor cycle time,
- proper chemicals,
- replenishment rate,
- temperatures (solutions and dryer),
- processor maintenance, and
- processor quality control (QC).

Figure 6–3 Standard and Extended Cycle Processes in Mammography. Characteristic curves are shown for a single-emulsion film recommended for mammography, using standard and extended-cycle processing. These curves show that an approximate 35% reduction in exposure may be achieved with the extended-cycle process without an increase in film fog.[9]

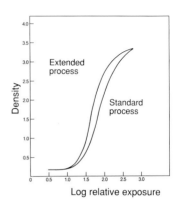

Processor Cycle Time

Processing time may be defined as the amount of time required for the leading edge of the film to enter and the trailing edge of the film to exit the processor. This is known as the *drop time*. Modern processing cycles range from approximately 45–210 seconds; although most automatic processors operate at 90 seconds for standard processing (**Figure 6–2a**). Film manufacturers determine optimal developer temperature and replenishment rates. These parameters are based on the processing cycle time required to achieve the desired sensitometric characteristics for the type of film being used.

Extended-cycle processing may be advantageous for some single-emulsion films. This method increases the length of *time* the film is in the developer while keeping the temperature essentially unchanged. For some single-emulsion films, specifically mammographic film, film contrast and speed are increased by extended-cycle processing without significantly affecting film fog (**Figure 6–3**). The increased speed permits a reduction in patient dose of approximately 35% when compared with equivalent density radiographs produced using the same screen-film combination and standard-cycle processing. Extended-cycle processing is not recommended for double-emulsion film.

Close inspection of **Figure 6–2b** reveals that the processing time (drop time) for extended-cycle processing is always longer than the time for standard processing for *the same model* film processor. Note, however, that by design, some processors with cycle times in excess of 90 seconds deliver "standard cycle" performance. Be sure to consult and maintain the film manufacturer's recommendations for time and temperature to achieve optimum processing, whether using standard or extended cycles.

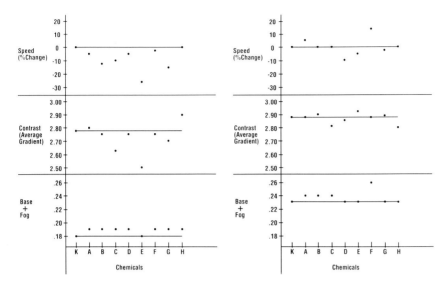

Figure 6–4 Film Processing Variations Due to Different Chemicals. Charts produced from film processing survey data that show film processing variations due to the use of different chemicals; data shown is for a single-emulsion film used for mammography **(left)** and a double-emulsion film used for conventional radiography **(right)**. The letter K indicates processing data (and expected values) using a Kodak processor and Kodak chemicals. A horizontal line begins above the letter K. Letters A through H are comparison data for different brands of chemicals. Data was obtained using film strips that were sensitometrically preexposed to light simulating the light spectrum from Kodak Lanex screens. Film speed differences, film contrast (average gradient), and base plus fog values were determined from the sensitometric data.[7]

Chemicals

All manufacturers recommend chemicals (or equivalents) and conditions (temperature, immersion times, replenishment rates) for processing their films. These factors have been tested by the manufacturers and have been shown to provide optimum processing. However, film speed, contrast, and base plus fog may vary when different chemicals are used for processing (**Figure 6–4**).

Processing chemical variability may occur because of a number of factors. Although most manufacturers use similar processing chemicals for development and fixation, the concentration of chemicals may vary either in the chemical concentrates produced by the manufacturer, or in the diluted end product mixed by on-site personnel or solution service providers. As a result, variations in concentration can produce suboptimal sensitometric characteristics of processed images.

Variability can also result from improper replenishment. Replenishment is important to maintain stable developer and fixer activity. Proper replenishment helps provide stable sensitometric results, minimizes artifacts, and promotes

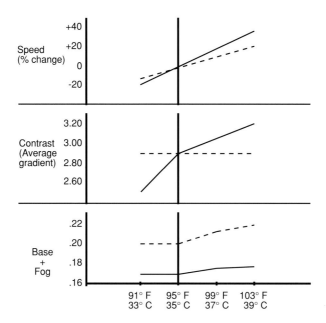

Figure 6–5 Effect of Developer Temperature on X-ray Film. Graph illustrating the effect of developer temperature on film speed, film contrast, and base plus fog. The percentage of film speed change, film contrast, and base plus fog are plotted vs the developer temperature for a single-emulsion, three-dimensional grain film (solid line), and a double-emulsion tabular grain film (dashed line). The vertical line represents the recommendation for a standard automatic processing cycle of 90 seconds.[7]

archival storage quality of processed radiographs. Replenishment rates are usually determined as a function of the amount of film processed per day (that is, total surface area or length of film). For example, 65 cc of developer replenishment may be required for each 14 in. x 17 in. film processed.

Lower volume processors that process few films per day require higher replenishment rates than high volume processors. It is very difficult to maintain the consistency of low volume processors, such as those in some operating rooms. A special replenishment technique, known as **flooded replenishment** or flood replenishment improves performance in these circumstances.[10] A starter solution is added to the developer replenisher holding tank. The processor is then replenished at specified time intervals.

For extended-cycle processing (mammography), especially close monitoring of replenishment is required for optimum results. Consult with the film manufacturer to correctly adjust and set up the film processor and replenishment rates required to obtain consistent, optimum results.

Temperature

Figure 6–5 illustrates the effect of developer temperature on sensitometric characteristics. Similar variations in results are to be expected with changes in development time.

Note that when the developer temperature is lower than the manufacturer's recommendation, film speed is reduced. As a result, an unnecessary increase in radiation dose will be required to produce radiographs of comparable optical density. Film contrast is also reduced when developer temperature is lowered. Conversely, if the developer temperature is higher or development time longer (extended-cycle process) than the film manufacturer's recommendation, film speed increases. This may permit a reduction in radiation dose and result in an increase in film contrast. However, these changes can usually be expected to increase radiographic noise (noise is discussed in Chapter 7). Increased developer temperature may also increase film fog. In addition, developer stability may be adversely affected when developer temperatures are used that are higher than those recommended by the manufacturer.

Preventive Maintenance

Automatic film processors are complex machines, combining chemical, mechanical, thermal, electrical, and often microcomputer-controlled systems. To maintain optimum processor performance, all of these systems must be operating within tolerances specified by the film manufacturer. Even deviations that seem insignificant, such as a one degree variation in developer temperature or a small non-uniformity on a cross-over roller, can cause unacceptable artifacts on processed images.

In order to maintain processor performance, the schedule of periodic preventive maintenance recommended by the manufacturer must be followed. In addition, processor cleaning and preventive maintenance checks must be performed by qualified individuals who have been trained in correct procedures for testing and repair.

One cannot think of an automatic film processor as an office copier that works in a darkroom. Although both machines have a sheet feeder and produce hard copy images, only radiographs from processors are used to diagnose disease in patients. To maintain the quality of processed radiographs, chemical and mechanical factors must be maintained within prescribed tolerances and monitored for consistency. Film processors require and deserve careful attention as an important component of patient care.

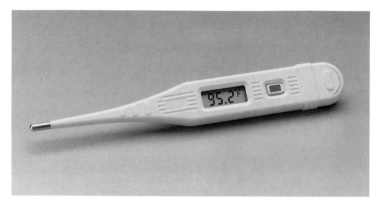

Figure 6–6 A Clinical, Digital Display Thermometer. This clinical, digital display thermometer, which may be used to monitor developer temperature in an automatic processor, has a temperature range of 90° to 108°F with an accuracy of plus or minus 0.2°F.[7]

PROCESSOR QUALITY CONTROL

Once the film processor has been adjusted for optimum performance, daily use has an effect on the parameters that control performance. In the normal course of operation, changes may occur in chemicals, temperature, the mechanics of the processor, or even the local water source used to supply the processor. Any one of these changes may cause enough of a degradation in processor performance to affect the quality of the processed images.

Different types of film can respond differently to processing variations. For example, a small change in processing conditions can significantly affect the film speed and contrast characteristics of single-emulsion mammography film, while having a minimal effect on double-emulsion tabular grain film used for general radiography. For ideal processor quality control, a facility should monitor the processor with each type of film processed in that processor.

A *daily* program of processor quality control is a fast, easy way to monitor the essential sensitometric properties of processed radiographs. Plotting these results provides immediate comparison with previously established operating limits of the processor. This enables the operator to detect drifts and to spot changes in performance and to make necessary corrections before clinical images have been adversely affected.

The four parameters monitored in a daily processor quality control (QC) program are developer temperature, speed index, contrast index, and base plus fog.

The National Council on Radiation Protection and Measurement (NCRP)

Report 99 on Quality Assurance[11], and the American College of Radiology (ACR) Mammography Quality Control Manual for Radiologic Technologists[12], indicate that the developer temperature should be within $\pm0.5°F$ ($\pm0.3°C$) of that recommended by the film manufacturer for the specific film-processing combination being used.

The measurement accuracy and precision of the thermometer are most important.* The thermometer used to measure developer temperature should have an accuracy at least equal to, or better than, the variability recommended in the NCRP and ACR documents. In radiology or medical imaging departments, a variety of thermometers may be used to measure developer temperature. These thermometers vary in accuracy, precision, ease of reading, and cost. A recent study suggests that clinical digital thermometers, which are available in pharmacies and supermarkets, are inexpensive but accurate devices for measuring developer solution temperature (**Figure 6–6**).[13] Thermometers used to measure developer temperature should also be evaluated against a thermometer that has a calibration traceable to the National Institute of Standards and Technology.

Monitoring of film contrast, film speed, and base plus fog values requires a sensitometer, densitometer, and a control chart (**Figure 6–7**).

A **sensitometer** is a device that is used in the darkroom to *expose* x-ray film to different light intensities in a "step" fashion. The color and range of brightnesses produced by the sensitometer simulate the range of light produced by the screens that expose film.

A **densitometer** is a device that is used to *measure the optical density* of selected steps after the exposed film has been processed. These results are then plotted on a **control chart**, which compares current with previous values of temperature, speed index, contrast index, and base plus fog. The control chart also indicates the control limits of these values. Results that fall on or outside the control limits indicate that corrective action is required.

Sample Procedure

Procedures for daily processor control are available from a number of sources, including film manufacturers and the American College of Radiology Mammography Accreditation Program. Although testing protocols differ somewhat in specific procedures, the following concepts are consistent.

1. Test film is exposed using a sensitometer and then processed.
2. Optical densities of particular steps are measured using a densitometer.
3. Key densities are compared and plotted against previously established values (**Figure 6–7**).

---

*Accuracy refers to the difference between the measured value and the value obtained from a standards laboratory. Precision refers to the degree of agreement of repeated measurements of a quantity.

Mammography Processing Control Chart

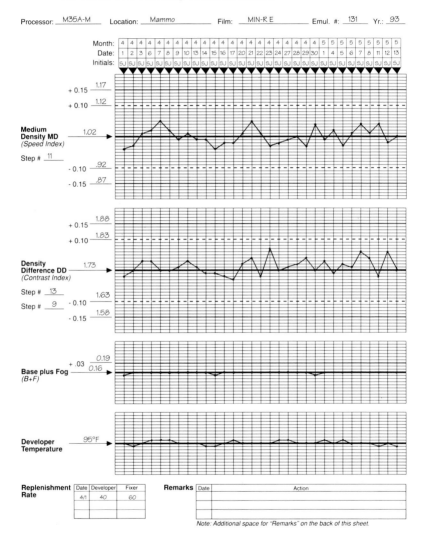

Figure 6–7 Processing Control Chart.   A processing control chart is used to record and monitor the following processor performance parameters: speed index, contrast index, base plus fog, and developer temperature. These parameters are measured daily and compared with preestablished values to help provide consistent processor performance.

4. Results are evaluated and, when necessary, corrective actions taken.

A sample procedure for mammography daily processor control is reproduced below.

Items Needed
1. Sensitometer with 21 density steps
2. Densitometer
3. Thermometer (**not** mercury) with an accuracy of $\pm 0.5°F$
4. Fresh box of 18 x 24 cm film, the same as that used for mammography
5. Control charts*

Establishing the Baseline
1. Ensure that:
   - the processor is thoroughly clean and functioning properly,
   - the processor is filled with properly mixed fresh chemicals,
   - the proper amount of developer starter has been added,
   - the proper developer temperature and replenishment rates have been set.
2. Set aside a fresh box of 18 x 24 cm film that is used for mammography. Designate it as your "QC" film and record the emulsion number on the control chart.
3. Set the sensitometer for the appropriate film spectral sensitivity (green for mammography) and either single- or double-emulsion film. (It is recommended that a sensitometer that exposes both film sides simultaneously be used for double-emulsion mammography film.)
4. On five (5) consecutive days, use film from the "QC" box to expose a sensitometric strip; process the film immediately. Note that:
   - the processor must be at the correct temperature,
   - the probe of the thermometer is consistently placed in the same area on the non-drive side of the processor developer tank,
   - single-emulsion film must be inserted into the sensitometer so the emulsion side faces the light-exposing source,
   - the sensitometric strip must be fed into the processor so that the less-exposed end is consistently fed first.
5. On the fifth day, use the densitometer to read the 21 density steps on each processed film. NOTE: Take the reading from the **middle** of each step.
6. Average the values of the 21 steps for the five days.

---

*Such as the "KODAK *Mammography Processing Control Chart*," publication number M7-173.

Determining Mid-Density (MD)

1. Determine which step has an average density closest to 1.20. Designate this step as the mid-density (MD) step for all future MD determinations and record the step number on the chart on the "Step #" line.
2. Write the average MD value on the arrow line following "Medium Density MD."

Determining Density Differences (DD)

1. Select the step with the average density closest to 2.20.
2. Select the step with the average density closest to, but not less than 0.45.
3. Subtract the density value determined in step 2 from the density value determined in step 1. This value will be the density difference (DD).
4. Designate the two steps as those to be used for all future DD determinations and record the step numbers on the chart on the two "Step #" lines. Write the average DD value on the arrow line following "Density Difference DD."

Determining Base + Fog

1. The five-day average of the least-exposed step (usually the first step) determines the Base + Fog of the film. (Any clear area of the film may also be used to determine Base + Fog.)
2. Write the average Base + Fog value on the arrow line following "Base plus Fog."

Developer Temperature

1. On the arrow line following "Developer Temperature," write the developer temperature recommended by the film manufacturer for your:
   • type of film,
   • developer (chemicals),
   • processor,
   • length of developer immersion time.

Establishing Operating Limits

1. The preferred mammography MD and DD operating limits are ± 0.10. The maximum outermost limits are ± 0.15.
2. Add 0.10 and 0.15 to the values on the arrow line for MD and DD; write the preferred and maximum **upper** limits after the respective +0.10 and +0.15 lines on the control chart.
3. Subtract 0.10 and 0.15 from the values on the arrow line for MD and DD; write the preferred and maximum **lower** limits after the respective –0.10 and –0.15 lines on the control chart.
4. Add 0.03 to the value on the arrow line for Base + Fog; write the **upper** limit on the control chart. (There is no lower limit for Base + Fog.)

Daily Processor Quality Control

1. Expose and process a sensitometric strip each morning that mammography films will be processed.
2. Select the same step numbers on the sensitometric strip that you recorded on your Mammography Processing Control Chart as the 5-day averages for MD and DD.
3. Use the densitometer to read the values for MD and DD, using the same steps recorded on the control chart.
4. Measure the Base + Fog. Use the first step or a clear area.
5. Plot the MD, DD, Base + Fog, and measured temperature values on the control chart.
6. Evaluate the results and make any necessary adjustments before processing any films.

Evaluating the Control Chart

1. Points that are plotted on the control chart for MD and DD that are within $\pm$ 0.10 should be considered normal process variations.
2. If any points are plotted on the control chart for MD and DD between $\pm$ 0.10 and $\pm$ 0.15, expose and process another sensitometric strip for comparison. Mammography films may be processed. The processor should be closely monitored to make certain that the outermost limits are not exceeded.
3. If any plotted points on the control chart for MD and DD reach or exceed $\pm$ 0.15, expose and process another sensitometric strip for comparison. If the same results are obtained, the American College of Radiology recommends that no mammography films be processed until the cause is determined and corrected. Plot the results obtained after the process has been brought back "in control." Note the action(s) taken to achieve this in the "Remarks" section on the control chart.
4. Any points plotted for Base + Fog that are within 0.03 are considered to be normal process variations; any points plotted for Base + Fog that exceed + 0.03 require immediate analysis.
5. The developer temperature should remain as close as possible to the temperature recommended by the film manufacturer; it should not vary by more that $\pm$ 0.5°F.
6. A trend exists if a series of consecutive points (three or more) progress steadily upward or downward. Such a trend may indicate a shift taking place slowly and visibly with respect to time. Monitor the processor closely.
7. Trends or gross fluctuations should be noted and evaluated. If necessary, appropriate action should be taken.
8. The "Remarks" section of the control chart should be used to note reasons for fluctuations such as routine preventive maintenance, fresh chemicals or the addition of developer starter.

The Crossover Procedure

When a new box of "QC" film is opened, perform the following **crossover procedure** to evaluate the characteristics of the new emulsion.

1. On the same day, at the same time, expose and immediately process five (5) sensitometric strips from the existing "QC" box and five (5) from the new "QC" box. NOTE: This procedure must be done when the chemicals are in a "seasoned," not a fresh state.

2. Using only the steps noted on the chart, determine the average values for MD, DD, and Base + Fog for the two groups of film.

3. Compare the values between the old and new boxes of film.
   - If the difference in MD and DD is > 0.05, change the operating level on the control chart (arrow line value) to the new number and note the reason for the change in the "Remarks" section.
   - If the difference in MD and DD is ≤ 0.05, either continue with the current values (ACR recommendations) or adjust the operating levels as when the difference is greater than 0.05.
   - If the average Base + Fog value for the new "QC" film is more than 0.02 higher than the old film, the reason for the increase must be determined.
   - Record the new emulsion number on the chart.

Final Comments

- It is recommended that a processor maintenance log be kept for each processor to record all service on the unit. This log can be used to correlate processor service with processor performance.
- The calibration of the sensitometer, densitometer, and thermometer should be checked periodically according to the recommendations, where available, of the film manufacturer.
- A Processing Control Chart may be used in various ways to monitor processor performance. For example, a new chart may be used for each month or information may be plotted continuously and a new chart started every 31 days.

RECOMMENDATIONS

1. Purchase processing systems from a reputable manufacturer that offers:
   - full-system product line,
   - service support,
   - technical support, and
   - educational support.

2. Follow the film manufacturer's recommendations for film processing and chemicals.

3. Implement a processor quality control program for routine monitoring of contrast, speed, base plus fog, and temperature.

SUMMARY

To obtain optimum film contrast and maximum film sensitivity (speed) in radiographs and medical images, it is essential to consider the film processor, film type, and chemicals as a total system. Film manufacturer's recommendations on processing for each type of radiographic or medical film used should always be followed. Most important, confirm and maintain film contrast, film speed (sensitivity), and film base plus fog values for film processor quality control.

Chapter 7
Radiographic Image Quality

Everyone wants quality images. Indeed, no one would deliberately choose poor quality images. The introduction to this volume identified this goal: to produce quality medical radiographic images at dose levels that are As Low As Reasonably Achievable (ALARA) for the betterment of patient care. While the concept of *image quality* is often used in a broad sense, it is valuable to understand the factors that contribute to image quality and the quantitative measurement of those factors.

The purpose of a radiographic image is to provide diagnostic information about a patient. In this text, the term *radiographic image quality* will be used as a description or quantitative measure of the excellence of an image with respect to the following components.

• Contrast
• Image blur
• Radiographic noise
• Artifacts

Note that the discussion of image quality has been confined to the technical aspects of a radiograph.

CONTRAST

This chapter begins with a review of the terms subject, film, and radiographic contrast and an investigation of the factors that affect each one, followed by a discussion of the interrelationship among all three types of contrast.

Subject Contrast

Subject contrast is the ratio of x-ray fluences emerging from two adjacent regions of the subject. It is a function of the pattern of x-ray fluences in the aerial image that expose the image receptor. Subject contrast depends upon factors that affect x-ray absorption in the subject (x-radiation beam spectrum and the nature of the subject) and upon scattered radiation (**Figure 7–1**).

Film Contrast

Film contrast is a measure of how differences in x-ray fluence, incident on the image receptor, will be converted into differences in optical density on a radiograph. Film contrast is the slope of the (film) characteristic curve. It is affected by film type, processing conditions used, density level in the radiograph, fog level of the film, and type of exposure (whether screen light or direct x ray) (**Figure 7–2**).

143

Factors Affecting Subject Contrast

Factor	Change	Subject Contrast
Beam spectrum		
kVp	↑	↓
Generator % ripple	↑	↑
Target material	W to Mo*	↑
Scatter		
kVp	↑	↓
Beam collimation (field size)	↑	↓
Grid or air-gap technique	Yes	↑
Compression	Yes	↑
Nature of subject		
Differences in x-ray absorption	↑	↑
Patient thickness	↑	↓
Arrows indicate increase (↑) or decrease (↓). *W-Tungsten, Mo-Molybdenum		

Figure 7–1 Factors Affecting Subject Contrast

Factors Affecting Film Contrast

Factor	Change	Film Contrast
Film type		
High contrast (short-scale)	Yes	↑
Wide latitude (long-scale)	Yes	↓
Position on film characteristic curve (density level)		
Toe		↓
Linear position		↑
Shoulder		↓
Fog level	↑	↓
Film processing		
Suboptimal	Yes	↓
Arrows indicate increase (↑) or decrease (↓).		

Figure 7–2 Factors Affecting Film Contrast

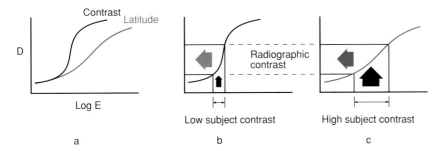

Figure 7–3 Radiographic Contrast. Radiographic contrast is the term used to describe the difference in optical density between two areas of interest in a radiograph. The slope of the characteristic curve is a measure of film contrast. **(a)** A wide-latitude film (red) can be used for long-scale imaging, such as chest radiography. **(b)** Low subject contrast in the aerial image may be imaged with a high-contrast film to produce good radiographic contrast. **(c)** Similar radiographic contrast may be obtained with high subject contrast in the aerial image and a latitude film.

Radiographic Contrast

Radiographic contrast is the term used to describe the difference in optical density between two areas of interest in a radiograph. Large differences in optical density indicate high radiographic contrast (short-scale). An image with high radiographic contrast is one in which regions on the film corresponding to areas of high x-ray absorption in the patient appear *very white*, while regions corresponding to areas of low x-ray absorption are *very dark*.

The components of radiographic contrast are subject contrast and film contrast. To clarify this relationship, consider the two sets of characteristic curves in **Figure 7–3a**. All characteristic curves may be thought of as describing the response or *output* of a system over a range of *input* conditions. A more familiar example to demonstrate the use of a characteristic curve might be a home audio system (**Figure 7–4**). The abscissa (x-axis) of the curve represents the input conditions, which in the case of the audio system is the volume setting on the amplifier. The ordinate (y-axis) represents the output—loudness of the two sets of speakers under comparison. The characteristic curves represent the response of the two sets of speakers (A and B). The loudness (output) is equal to the volume control setting (input), multiplied by the response characteristic curve of the respective speaker.

In the context of radiographic imaging, **Figure 7–3a** describes the now familiar film characteristic curve. In this case, the *input* is the different x-ray fluences within the aerial image that strike the image receptor, that is, the subject contrast along the Log E axis. The characteristic curves represent the response of two screen-film systems, A and B, the slope of which is the film contrast. The *output* of the radiographic system is the optical density produced on the film. For

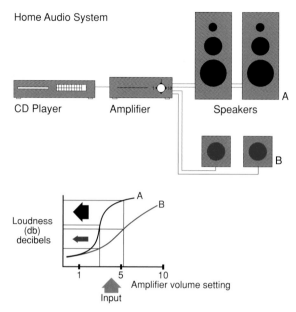

Figure 7–4 Home Audio System and Characteristic Curves. A characteristic curve describes the output of a system over a range of input conditions. The home audio system has two sets of speakers (top, A and B) and two sets of charactertistic curves (bottom, A and B). The input to the speakers is the range of amplifier volume settings (x-axis). The output of the speakers is the loudness, shown on the y-axis. The output is equal to the volume setting (input) multiplied by the characteristic curve for each set of speakers. Note that the A speakers provide more output (loudness) than the B speakers for the same amplifier volume setting.

a given screen-film system, the difference in optical density is the radiographic contrast.

Consider the effects of different subject and film contrast on radiographic contrast, as shown in **Figure 7–3**. In **Figure 7–3b**, the input or subject contrast is low, due to the high kVp needed on a portable exam (non-grid) to penetrate a thick body part. A high-contrast, screen-film system may be used to provide high radiographic contrast (output). In **Figure 7–3c**, the subject contrast is increased but film contrast is reduced. This could have been caused by performing the same exam at a lower kVp in the imaging department with a grid (increased subject contrast), but with the inadvertent use of a chest cassette loaded with wide-latitude film (decreased film contrast, long-scale). The result is comparable output, that is, radiographic contrast. In the first exam, the lower subject contrast input has been somewhat compensated for by the use of a high-contrast, screen-film system.

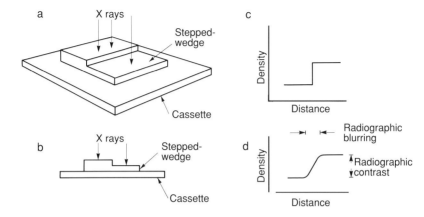

Figure 7–5 The Effect of Radiographic Contrast and Blur on Radiographic Sharpness. **(a and b)** A stepped-wedge with a sharp, vertical boundary between steps is exposed to x rays. **(c)** A plot of (optical) density readings that would be expected across the resulting radiograph if there were no image blur (perfect system) is shown. The densities are read in a direction perpendicular to the boundaries between the steps, with the lower density occurring under the thicker step. This ideal, sharp screen-film image never occurs in practice. A density trace across the stepped-wedge image shows the effect of image blur and radiographic contrast. **(d)** Because of geometric blurring and light diffusion, the optical density change represented by the boundary between the steps has a gradual slope, compared with the steep rise of the perfect system (c).

IMAGE BLUR

An image may be said to have high detail if it exhibits minimum unsharpness. In this text, the concept of **image blur** will continue to be emphasized. In theory, an infinitesimally small object (a "point") can produce an infinitesimally small image. In radiography, this is not possible due to the presence of blur in the imaging system.[4] The amount of image blur may be quantified by imaging a point object and measuring its size on a radiograph.

Other terms are used to describe this phenomenon in a subjective manner, for example, radiographic sharpness, which is the subjective impression of the distinctness or perceptibility of the boundary or edge of a structure in a radiograph. Radiographic sharpness is related to the magnitude and width, that is, the abruptness of the density change across the boundary (**Figure 7–5**).

A test device, commonly called a **bar pattern,** is used to quantify the amount of blur in an image. A bar pattern is made from a series of metal strips. The width of each strip (and corresponding spaces) decreases along the length of the test device. At first glance, a radiograph of a bar pattern (**Figure 7–6a**) might seem to provide an ideal, quantitative measure of image blur. For example, if the strips and

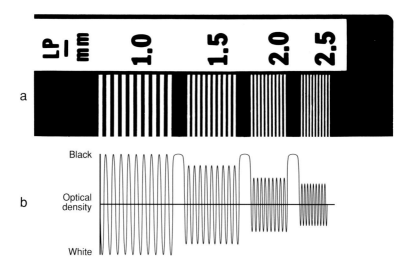

Figure 7–6 A Bar Resolution Test Pattern. **(a)** A radiograph of a bar pattern made from a series of metal strips with decreasing thickness and separation is shown. (Courtesy of Nuclear Associates, Carle Place, NY). **(b)** A microdensitometer trace shows the effect on optical density (radiographic contrast) as the line spacing decreases. Radiographic contrast is the difference in these optical densities.

spacers can be clearly seen down to 2.5 line pairs (lp) per mm, it could be said that the system is capable of a 2.5 lp/mm resolution.

While conceptually straightforward and somewhat intuitively satisfying, several problems limit the usefulness of this approach.

1. The point at which the image of the strips and spacers becomes blurred requires a subjective determination. Different observers have different judgments of which strips are blurred. Consequently, this method is not very reproducible.

2. The test pattern provides some information about the size of the metal strips that may be seen in a radiograph. In medical radiography, however, the goal is to image fundamentally different kinds of objects.

3. The bar pattern image in **Figure 7–6a** may be evaluated using a scanning microdensitometer. This device plots the optical densities of a continuous series of small points across the film. Note the decrease in radiographic contrast between images of strips, and spacers, as their widths decrease (**Figure 7–6b**). A connection exists between radiographic contrast and the ability to perceive distinct strips and spacers in the image that is not addressed by a simple description of which lines are or are not resolved.

Another method describes image blur in a more precise, practical, and observer-independent manner. Consider the experiment in **Figure 7–7**. Blur was previously defined in terms of the image of a point-object. (A basic geometric principle states that the width of a line is the width of a point.) This experiment

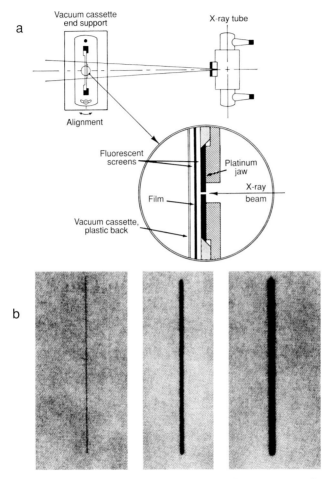

Figure 7–7 Slit Images. **(a)** Diagram of an apparatus used to make x-ray slit exposures for line spread function (LSF) measurements.[14] **(b)** Screen-film radiographs of a slit using the same film. The width of the slit image increases from left to right as screens of increasing thickness are used. This demonstrates the effect of screen thickness on image blur.[15]

---

investigates the characteristics of the *image of the line* produced by a slit test object. A plot of a microdensitometer scan of the image is known as the **line spread function** (**Figure 7–8**).

To derive more general information than can be provided by the line spread function, a powerful mathematical tool—the **Fourier transform**—is applied to the line spread function. The result is the **modulation transfer function**. Appendix C provides an intuitive understanding of the Fourier transform and modulation transfer function.

a
b

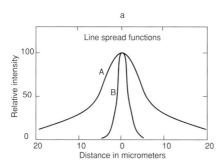
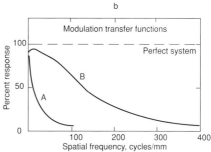

Figure 7–8 Line Spread Function and Modulation Transfer Function. **(Left)** A microdensitometer scan of a 10 μm-wide slit image (radiograph) using a thick screen (A) and a thin screen (B) appear. These are called line spread functions (LSFs). **(Right)** The modulation transfer function (MTF) is the Fourier Transform of the line spread function. The MTFs corresponding to the thick and thin screens (A and B) are shown; the MTF of a perfect system is shown for reference.

Radiographic Blur

The components of radiographic contrast are subject contrast and film contrast. Similarly, those factors in the summary charts of **Figures 7–1** and **7–2** that cause an increase in subject and film contrast (radiographic contrast) also cause perceptibility of the boundary to improve. That is, they improve radiographic sharpness. In other words, as the density difference between the steps increases, visibility of the edge improves and sharpness increases, if other factors remain unchanged.

The three radiographs of a bone specimen shown in **Figure 7–9** also demonstrate the effects of radiographic contrast and radiographic blur on the image. **Figure 7–9a** was made with a screen, which produces considerable image blur because of its thickness. Even though it has high contrast, this radiograph exhibits increased image blur because of the lateral spreading of the light within the screen-film combination. **Figure 7–9b**, made without screens, shows minimal image blur. However, the film contrast is low (**Figure 7–9b**), which tends to offset the gain from reduced image blur. The result is that sharpness is less than optimal. **Figure 7–9c** was made with screens that had a thin phosphor layer containing a light-absorbing dye, thereby reducing image blur from light diffusion. This effect, combined with high film contrast, produces an image with boundaries that are more distinct (reduced image blur) than the other two radiographs.

Radiographic Noise

Unwanted variations in the optical density across a radiograph impair the ability to distinguish objects. When these variations in density are random, they

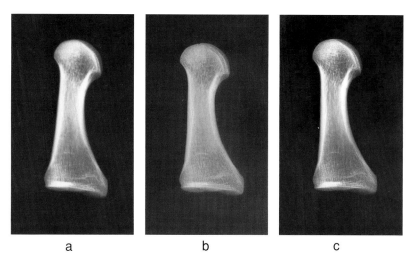

a   b   c

Figure 7–9 Radiographic Contrast and Image Blur. **(a)** Radiograph of a bone specimen made with a screen-film combination that produces considerable image blur. Note that even though the radiographic contrast is high, the image is not sharp. **(b)** A direct exposure radiograph made without intensifying screens exhibits minimal blur. The low film contrast impairs the perceptibility of detail in the image. **(c)** A radiograph made with thin screens containing a light-absorbing dye to reduce light diffusion is combined with a high-contrast film. This reduction in image blur improves the perceptibility of detail when compared with a and b.

are collectively described as **radiographic noise**. In radio or TV broadcasting, the term noise is frequently used to describe the sound or image from a weak signal. In these cases, random variations caused by inadequate signal strength produce the scratchy sounds (radio) and speckled images (TV) that are described as "noisy." Noise produces a similar effect in radiography.

Radiographic Mottle

Radiographic mottle is the density variation in a radiograph made with intensifying screens that have been exposed to uniform x-radiation fluence. It consists of three components: structure mottle, film graininess, and quantum mottle.

Structure mottle is the density fluctuation resulting from non-uniformity in the structure of intensifying screens. Inhomogeneities in the phosphor layer, such as clumping of the phosphor crystals or coating variations, would result in varying amounts of screen light output and therefore film density fluctuations. However, in most commercially available screens, structure mottle is not a practical problem. The combined effect of structure mottle and quantum mottle (described later in this chapter) is sometimes referred to as **screen mottle**.

Film graininess is the visual impression of the density variation (granularity) in a film exposed to a uniform fluence of light. In this case, the exposing light

a   b

Figure 7–10 Radiograph of Mottle vs Film Granularity. **(a)** This image was produced using a screen-film combination that was given a uniform x-ray exposure. The irregular pattern of optical densities is due primarily to quantum mottle. **(b)** A second image was produced by uniform exposure of the film to light alone (without screens). The noise in this image is due to film granularity.

does not arise from intensifying screens because exposure by intensifying screens produces quantum mottle, which overwhelms any film graininess. Film granularity is due to the random distribution of deposits of developed silver. **Figure 7–10b** shows the pattern produced on x-ray film by uniform exposure to light alone. Notice how much smoother it appears than the pattern of radiographic mottle shown in **Figure 7–10a**, which was made with intensifying screens. The density fluctuations in **Figure 7–10a** are due almost exclusively to quantum mottle, since the other two components, structure mottle and film graininess, make an insignificant contribution to this pattern.

The following discussion about the insignificance of film graininess relative to quantum mottle is generally true for radiographs as normally viewed on a viewbox. However, in cases where a portion of the radiograph is magnified by a lens or by projection on a screen, film graininess can be seen, particularly for low-density areas.

QUANTUM MOTTLE

The effect of a *limited* number of x-ray photons (or quanta) on the appearance of the radiograph is called *quantum mottle*, and is the major contributor to image noise. This mottled image is due to insufficient x-ray photons. This effect is similar to the phenomenon we experience when we try to see under low-light conditions (insufficient light photons). If you turn off the room lights and allow a few moments to dark-adapt, you will be able to see some image detail, but will notice a mottled appearance to the visual image. This effect is analogous to that which is observed in an image owing to insufficient x-ray photons in a radiograph.[16]

Quantum mottle is seen as the variation in density of a radiograph exposed to a uniform fluence of x-ray photons, which results from the *random spatial*

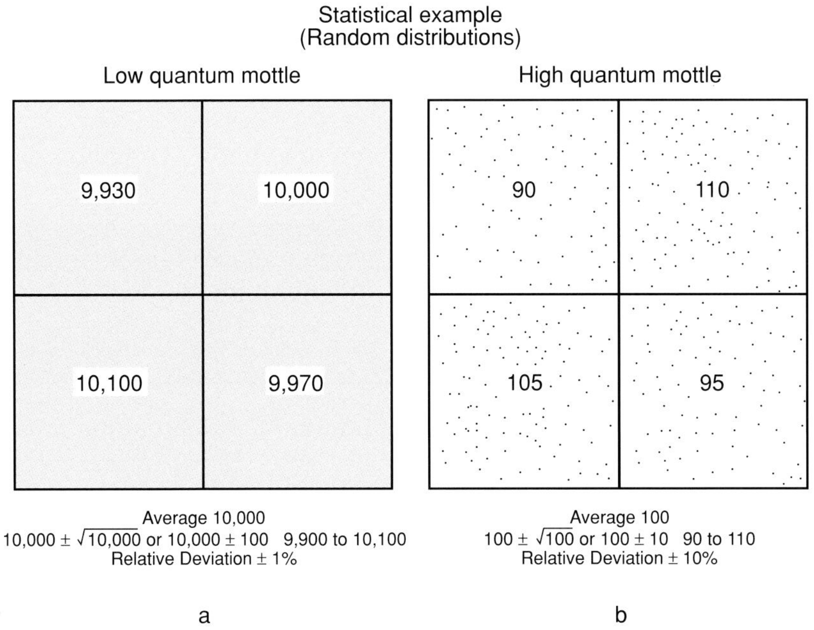

Statistical example
(Random distributions)

Low quantum mottle   High quantum mottle

9,930	10,000
10,100	9,970

Average 10,000
$10,000 \pm \sqrt{10,000}$ or $10,000 \pm 100$ 9,900 to 10,100
Relative Deviation $\pm 1\%$

90	110
105	95

Average 100
$100 \pm \sqrt{100}$ or 100 ± 10 90 to 110
Relative Deviation $\pm 10\%$

a   b

Figure 7–11 Water Droplet Analogy. In radiography, quantum mottle is related to the square root of the total number of x-ray absorption events in an image receptor. **(a)** In this analogy, a bucket with 40,000 water droplets is poured over four concrete squares to demonstrate low quantum mottle. **(b)** To demonstrate increased quantum mottle, the number of water droplets has been reduced to 400. Note that the relative deviation in the low quantum mottle scenario (a) is $\pm 1\%$ compared with $\pm 10\%$ with high quantum mottle (b).

distribution of the x-ray quanta absorbed in the screen. For a given intensifying screen and optical density level, as the number of x-ray absorption events in the screen decreases, the quantum mottle (noise) increases. The following analogy may help to clarify this concept.

Water Droplet Analogy

Consider four square sections in a concrete sidewalk and a bucket of water about to be emptied over the four squares (**Figure 7–11**). The concrete squares correspond to the screen-film combination and the water droplets to the x-ray photons absorbed by the screens to produce light. The bucket contains 40,000 water droplets. (Note that this is not the same as the number of x-ray photons *incident* on the screen, because only those absorbed by the screen phosphors generate light to produce the radiographic image.) The wetness of the sidewalk is analogous to the optical density of the radiograph.

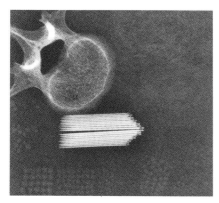 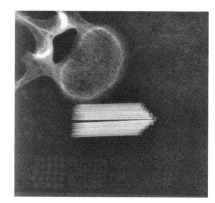

Figure 7–12 The Effect of Screen-Film Contact on Quantum Mottle and Radiographic Sharpness. **(Left)** A radiograph made with screens and film in close contact is compared with **(right)** an image made with screens separated from the film by a sheet of clear acetate. Poor screen-film contact produces image blur, which reduces visualization of the quantum mottle. Image resolution is also reduced.

When the bucket is overturned, suppose that an average of 10,000 droplets fall on each square of sidewalk. Since water droplets fall at random, the actual number that fall on each square is not exactly 10,000 per square, but varies slightly from this number. Mathematical methods may be used to predict the outcome of a random process (for example, Poisson statistics, which are described in textbooks on statistics). For this discussion, however, numbers that are both mathematically correct and intuitively acceptable will be used, without discussing the underlying statistical theory. In this example, there will be some small difference in the number of drops that fall on each of the four squares. Therefore, if this experiment were repeated several times, the actual number of droplets to fall on each square would most probably be a little different each time. This variation in the number of water droplets is due to the statistical fluctuations of random events in nature, which correspond to variations in the number of x-ray quanta absorbed in an intensifying screen.

Now imagine that the bucket is filled with only 400 water droplets. When overturned, each concrete block will be exposed to approximately 100 droplets. At the same time, suppose that the concrete has been treated with a special substance, which results in the *same* degree of wetness (optical density) from approximately 100 drops per square as that in the original concrete blocks with 10,000 drops each. In radiography, this would be analogous to using a faster film, which requires less screen light exposure to produce the same optical density as a normal speed film.

Upon comparing the appearance of the two sets of concrete blocks, note that the untreated blocks exposed to about 10,000 droplets each have a much more uniformly wet appearance than do the specially treated blocks. Those blocks exposed to the fewer number of droplets exhibit a more blotchy appearance. Radiographs exposed using the analogous faster film would present a similar blotchy, mottled appearance when compared with those exposed using a slower film. The screen-film combination using the slower film required more x-ray absorption events to produce a given optical density. Therefore, quantum mottle was reduced when compared with the use of a faster film and the same intensifying screen. Conversely, use of a faster film increases system speed (that is, less radiation exposure is required to produce a given optical density) at a cost of increased quantum mottle.

System speed can also be increased by holding the film speed constant and increasing the screen speed. Higher speed screens absorb a higher portion of x-ray photons from the incident beam by using more phosphor material. This may be accomplished by changing from one to two screens in a cassette (along with double-emulsion film), increasing screen thickness, or increasing the packing density of phosphors within the screen. The number of x-ray absorption events in the screen is thereby increased to increase system speed, and quantum mottle is not noticeably affected. Wherever possible, increasing screen speed is the preferred method of increasing system speed.

Factors Affecting the Visibility of Quantum Mottle

Every screen-film image contains a certain degree of quantum mottle. When quantum mottle is very visible, it interferes with our ability to interpret radiographs, particularly small, low-contrast objects in the image (**Figure 7–12**). The negative impact of quantum mottle in an image is affected by both the amount and visibility of the mottle, as influenced by the following factors.

1. **Film Speed** If film speed is increased, fewer x-ray quanta are needed to produce a given density in the radiograph and quantum mottle increases. Conversely, a slower film offers one way of reducing quantum mottle.

2. **Film Contrast** As film contrast increases, visibility of quantum mottle increases. A high-contrast film produces a larger density difference in the radiograph than does a low-contrast film for a given variation in log relative exposure. This occurs whether the log relative exposure differences are the result of subject contrast or quantum mottle. Accordingly, quantum mottle is more visible in a high-contrast film than in a low-contrast film.

3. **Screen Conversion Efficiency** As screen conversion efficiency increases, quantum mottle increases. Screen conversion efficiency is the ratio of light energy emitted by the screen to the x-ray energy absorbed in it. A more efficient phosphor produces more light for each x-ray quantum absorbed and therefore fewer x-ray quanta are needed to produce a given density in the radiograph than that required for a less efficient phosphor. As the number of quanta used to produce a given density decreases, quantum mottle increases.

4. **Absorption** Changing the thickness of the phosphor layer or changing to a phosphor with different absorption characteristics alters the absorption of x-ray quanta in the screen. However, we know that as screen thickness increases, screen blur also increases. The combination of these effects is such that a thicker screen may produce more quantum mottle, but the increased screen blur makes the mottle less visible. As a result, the appearance of quantum mottle in the radiograph may not be appreciably altered, although overall image blur would increase, thereby reducing image quality. Minimal quantum mottle in a fast screen-film combination is indicative of increased image blur introduced by the screen.

Conversely, if x-ray absorption is increased by changing to a phosphor having greater absorption without a change in screen thickness, then image blur and quantum mottle will be the same as for the less absorbing screen. Of course, patient exposure could be reduced to provide radiographs of equivalent optical density. Remember that it is the number of *absorbed* x-ray quanta, not incident quanta, that controls the amount of quantum mottle.

5. **Radiation Quality** When the x-ray beam is made "harder," that is, when the average energy of the photons in the beam is increased by raising kVp, the average energy of the x-ray quanta absorbed by the screen is increased. The greater the energy of each photon, the brighter the screen light (the greater the number of light photons) emitted when the x-ray photon is absorbed. The brighter screen light emission implies that fewer x-ray photons will be required to produce a given film density. For this reason, the use of higher kVp increases quantum mottle somewhat.

Effect of Quantum Mottle on Image Quality

Quantum mottle can affect the visibility of structures in a radiograph. For example, compare the images of the beads in **Figure 7–13**. Many more x-ray quanta (more x-ray absorption events) were required to produce the radiograph in **Figure 7–13a** than in **Figure 7–13b**. Consequently, the increased quantum mottle in **Figure 7–13b** has noticeably degraded the image quality. Quantum mottle has a relatively greater effect on the perceptibility of low-contrast objects, such as cysts or soft-tissue lesions.

ARTIFACTS

Artifacts are unwanted density variations in the form of blemishes in the radiograph that arise from improper handling, exposure, processing or housekeeping. Appendix D discusses a number of artifact causes. Some artifacts, such as those produced from dirty film processor rollers, produce images with a "mottled" appearance. These artifacts are not, however, due to random statistical fluctuations and therefore are not representative of quantum mottle.

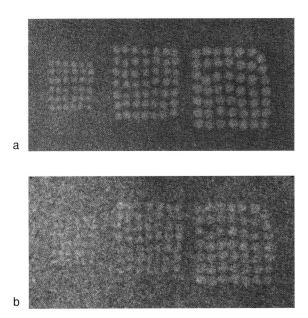

Figure 7–13 Effect of Quantum Mottle on Image Quality. **(a)** A radiograph of a phantom containing moderate absorbing beads made with a slow screen-film combination using many x-ray quanta (low quantum mottle) is compared with **(b)** a radiograph made with a fast screen-film combination using relatively few x-ray quanta (high quantum mottle).

VIEWING CONDITIONS

Much of the information contained in the radiographic image cannot be seen if proper consideration is not given to viewing conditions. Radiographs should be interpreted under conditions that provide good visibility, comfort, and minimal fatigue.

The illuminator surface should provide diffused light of uniform brightness and variations in surface luminance should be gradual. The luminance level must be sufficient to illuminate areas of interest in the radiograph. Ideally, all viewboxes should have lamps of the same color.

The contrast sensitivity of the eye (the ability to distinguish small luminance differences) is greatest when surroundings are of about the same brightness as the area of interest. Therefore, to see detail in a radiograph, it is important to reduce glare to a minimum, to avoid surface reflections, and to reduce ambient light level to approximately that reaching the eye through the radiograph. Glare and reflections can be reduced by locating illuminators away from bright surroundings such as windows, by turning off surrounding viewboxes when not in use, and by using masks to cover unused portions of a viewbox or to cover

Contrast		Blur		Noise	Artifacts
Subject Contrast	Film Contrast	Geometric Blur	Light Diffusion		
Absorption differences in subject Thickness Density Atomic number Contrast media	Film type Processing Solution activity Formulation Mixing Replenishment Contamination Oxidation	Focal spot size Focal-object distance Object-film distance	Screens Phosphor thickness Reflector Light absorbing dyes and pigments Phospor particle size	Quantum mottle Film speed Film contrast Screen conversion efficiency Screen absorption Radiation quality Light diffusion	Handling Crimp marks Fingerprints Scratches Static
Radiation quality Kilovoltage Voltage waveform Target material	Temperature Time Agitation	Motion Patient Equipment	Film Crossover	Structure mottle	Exposure Fog Light leaks Spilled contrast media
Scattered radiation Beam limitation Grids Air gap Compression	Optical density Fog Storage Safelight Light leaks		Screen-film contact	Film graininess	Processing Streaks Spots Drying Contamination Scratches Deposits
Extra-focal radiation	Exposure type Screen Direct				Screens and film Dirt Stains

Figure 7–14 Factors Affecting Radiographic Image Quality

low-density areas in the radiograph being examined.

Subdued lighting is preferred in the viewing room. It is also convenient to have available a variable high-output light source (with appropriate masks) to view high-density areas on radiographs, as well as reducing or magnifying glasses for examining certain types of structures.

SUMMARY

Many factors contribute to the quality (excellence) of a radiograph. **Figure 7–14** summarizes many of these factors. Image quality requirements vary with different clinical requirements. For example, one might assume that a slower screen-film combination that minimizes noise and produces a sharp image of a stationary subject would be most desirable. However, for some examinations, the image resulting from such a combination may be less useful than one produced with a faster screen-film combination having more quantum mottle and less sharpness. The faster combination may provide more diagnostic information because of its ability to arrest motion by permitting shorter exposure times, to increase subject contrast by allowing the use of a lower kVp, or to give a magnified image by enabling the use of a smaller focal spot and increased distance.

It might seem that high contrast is always desirable because it tends to increase sharpness. However, if latitude is insufficient because contrast is too high, structures of interest may not be visualized, requiring repeat exposures.

Our understanding of the relationships among the factors affecting radiographic image quality is still evolving. Choices of exposure conditions and recording materials must be based on experience, taking into account the imaging task (the examination to be performed) and the needs of the person interpreting the image. The selection of appropriate image quality factors will always involve compromises. The more we understand the interaction between these factors, the better the contribution we can make to producing radiographic images of high quality.

Chapter 8

Recording Electronic Digital Images

All medical imaging techniques, whether conventional radiography or the most sophisticated digital imaging systems, use similar approaches to the three basic phases of the imaging cycle:

1. **Produce the aerial image**—All techniques must optimize differences in x-ray absorption between structures of interest and surrounding tissue. That is, all must produce an aerial image with the best characteristics to meet a specific diagnostic need.

2. **Capture and display the aerial image** —Since the human observer cannot see the aerial image, it must be altered to permit viewing and interpretation of the information. The use of phosphors to convert the x-ray energy of the aerial image into a more usable form is common to all medical radiography except direct exposure technique. The display characteristics of the image must also be optimized to meet specific clinical needs.

3. **Record and archive the visual image**—The image must be recorded in such a manner as to enable ease of viewing, ease of comparison with results of other imaging modalities, and ease of transfer to other locations (both near and far), and ultimately, archival storage for later retrieval.

ANALOG VS DIGITAL IMAGES

In conventional systems, the operator selects the technique factors to optimize subject contrast, image blur, and noise in the aerial image. The second and third phases of the imaging cycle use a screen-film combination. Intensifying screens (with phosphors) convert the x-ray energy of the aerial image into light energy, which exposes sensitized radiographic film and forms the latent image. The brightness of screen light emitted varies in a continuous manner, with proportionately more light emitted by regions of the screen that have been exposed to greater x-ray fluences. The proportionality of screen light emitted is transferred to the x-ray film, producing proportionately greater film blackening with increasing screen light exposure. Such a system is said to be an *analog* system because the image capture and recording phases make use of the continuously variable signals.

In the capture phase, the signal refers to the screen light output, which is continuously variable (light rays) and proportional to the x-ray photon fluence in the aerial image. In the final phase, the light from the fluorescent screens is recorded on silver halide film in a continuous gray scale. **Figure 8–1** illustrates the differences between *analog* and *digital* signals and images as they apply in fluoroscopy.

The display characteristics of the image are controlled by selecting an image receptor with film contrast, blur, and noise characteristics to meet specified imaging requirements. Film processing brings these specific characteristics "into

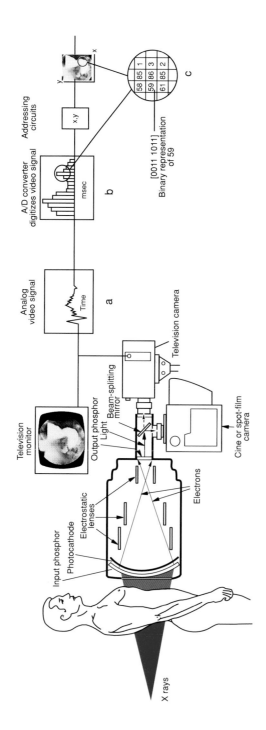

Figure 8–1 Analog and Digital Signals in Fluoroscopy. The video signal from the television camera is analog, where the voltage signal varies continuously. (**a**) This analog signal is sampled, producing (**b**) a stepped representation of the analog video signal. (**c**) The numerical values of each step are stored, producing a matrix of digital image data. The binary representation of each pixel value in the matrix is stored and can be manipulated by a computer. The value of each pixel can be mapped to a brightness level for viewing on a CRT, or to an optical density for hard copy on film.

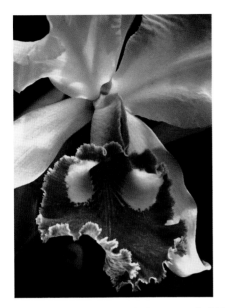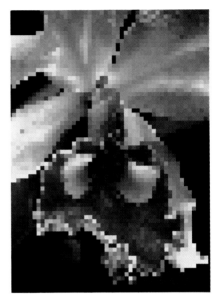

Figure 8–2 Analog vs Digital Images. **(Left)** In an analog image (conventional photograph), the shades of gray vary continuously. The film grain is imperceptibly small. **(Right)** A finite number of shades of gray and the noticeable size of each pixel have been exaggerated to demonstrate the digitized representation of the same image.

view" in the finished radiograph. A transportable, archival record is produced that possesses the information contained in the aerial image and displays the image along with the radiographic contrast, blur, and noise characteristics of the screen-film system.

Electronic imaging systems differ from screen-film techniques in that the conversion of x-ray energy in the aerial image is accomplished using a medium other than an intensifying screen. Electronic images are displayed using cathode ray tubes (CRTs), which may display either analog video or digital images (**Figure 8–2**). In analog video fluoroscopy, the video camera (tube) produces an electronic signal of continuously varying voltages, which is used to stimulate the brightness of the phosphor of the CRT.

The word *pixel* is a commonly used abbreviation for *pic*ture *el*ement. A pixel refers to the smallest unit in the image matrix, a point with a specific coordinate (row and column location) corresponding to a location in the patient. The location *in the patient* that corresponds to a pixel is called a *voxel*, or *vo*lume *el*ement. To help remember the distinction, recall that only patients have volume, hence *voxel*. Digital images are pictures made up of *pixels*. The value of each pixel is the digital representation of the characteristic (or parameter) measured by each modality (for example, computed tomography and magnetic resonance) to form an image. For example, in digital fluoroscopy, the image parameter represented by the pixel is the x-ray fluence in the aerial image. An ultrasound image pixel represents the strength of the sound wave echo detected by the transducer. The radio-frequency (RF) signal strength is the image parameter detected by the coils in a magnetic resonance imaging system.

These systems are *digital* because the image information is carried in the form of *bi*nary digi*ts* (bits), with sampled values of the imaging parameter. A bit can have a value of either 0 or 1, representing electrical signals that have only two states, such as "on" or "off," or "high" or "low" voltages. The terms binary and digital are used interchangeably. Since digital signals are binary (that is, separate or discrete values of energy), they are said to be non-continuous, as opposed to analog (continuous) signals.

In some cases, electronic image data may be temporarily or permanently stored using magnetic or optical disk technology. Essentially all electronic imaging systems can utilize the advantages of silver halide film for image archive and transfer.

Electronic images are transferred to film by the use of a laser imaging device. In this context, electronic imaging systems will be briefly described, followed by a review of the laser imager.

FLUOROSCOPY

By far, the most common electronic x-ray imaging technique is **fluoroscopy**, which uses an image intensifier tube to convert the x-ray energy of the aerial image into a minified, visible light image (**Figure 8–1**). In conventional fluoroscopy, a video tube converts the visible light image into an analog video signal that can be viewed on a TV monitor and stored on video tape or video disk. Fluoroscopic systems offer the capability of real-time imaging, creating a moving picture of dynamic function within the patient. The visible light image may also be imaged onto light-sensitive film to produce spot films or cineradiography. These techniques use the high resolution characteristics of film to produce hard copy images with superior image detail, compared with that of either analog or digital electronic fluoroscopic imaging.

Digital fluoroscopic systems convert the analog video signal into digital data. The result is a matrix of digital data for each video frame, corresponding to the brightness of the visible light characteristics of the image. The digital image consists of rows and columns of data, each individual "point" being called a pixel.

COMPUTED TOMOGRAPHY

Computed tomography (CT) scanners create digital images by measuring the transmission of an x-ray beam through tissue as the x-ray tube rotates around the patient. Hundreds to thousands of x-ray detectors (usually solid-state detectors) measure the attenuation of the fan-shaped x-ray beam by structures within the patient. These detectors collect the information from each projection. The information is digitized and analyzed by a computer to reconstruct cross-sectional CT images. CT imaging offers many diagnostic advantages, including the ability to produce reconstructed images in selected projections, as well as low-contrast resolution far superior to that of all other x-ray imaging modalities.

NUCLEAR IMAGING

Nuclear imaging enables radioactive materials to be chemically attached to physiologically significant compounds to produce images that document function and flow within the body. Radioactively tagged compounds are injected into, or are ingested by, the patient. These labeled compounds are preferentially absorbed by their respective target organs, resulting in increased radioactivity corresponding to the function of the organ of interest. The Anger Scintillation Camera, commonly known as a *gamma camera*, uses a sodium iodide crystal to absorb gamma rays emanating from the patient. When a gamma ray photon is absorbed, a flash of light is produced in the crystal and detected by an array of photomultiplier tubes (PMTs). Electric signals produced by the PMTs are processed to create an image on a CRT. Most systems use a camera to transfer the CRT images to film. The digital image may be manipulated by any number of image processing techniques to aid in diagnosis. The ability of these images to convey information about both structure and function has created a unique and valuable niche for nuclear imaging.

MAGNETIC RESONANCE IMAGING

Magnetic resonance (MR) scanners utilize a magnetic field and radio frequency (RF) instead of ionizing radiation to create digital images. Key elements in the body—especially hydrogen—will respond to magnetic fields and RF energy with a characteristic resonance phenomenon. The MR scanner detects these resonances and produces electrical signals that are processed to construct images in multiple planes, such as coronal and sagittal planes.

While MR images appear to resemble CT images, MR images are based on properties that are fundamentally different from the x-ray absorption characteristics that provide contrast in CT imaging.

ULTRASOUND IMAGING

Non-ionizing radiation such as **ultrasound** may be used to provide diagnostic electronic images. An ultrasound transducer generates pulses of sound waves with frequencies well beyond the limit of human hearing. Ultrasound waves are transmitted through and reflected by anatomic structures in their path. The transducer also detects the reflected waves, producing an electronic image on a CRT with a brightness corresponding to the strength of the ultrasound echoes. Ultrasound imaging does not use ionizing radiation and it has the ability to distinguish between solid masses and cysts. For these reasons, it has become an indispensable imaging tool.

DIGITAL RADIOGRAPHY USING STORAGE PHOSPHORS

Digital or **computed radiography** (CR) describes techniques that capture the information in the aerial image using storage phosphors. **Storage phosphor screens** look very much like and perform similarly to conventional intensifying screens, storing information in the latent image for later *read out* and display.[17]

Depending on the screen phosphor material, the latent image signal remains stable for a period of time (from minutes to days) before it decays to a level at which image quality will be adversely affected. The latent image can be *read out* with a scanning system and displayed on a CRT.

A storage phosphor latent image is *read out* using a red or near-infrared light to stimulate the phosphor, causing it to release its stored energy in the form of visible light (**Figure 8–3**). This phenomenon is known as *photostimulable luminescence*. As with conventional intensifying screens, the intensity of this stimulated luminescence is proportional to the number of x-ray photons absorbed by the storage phosphor.

Rather than flood the surface of the screen with stimulating light, the *read-out* process is accomplished using a laser scanner. The laser beam scans the surface of the screen in a raster pattern similar to the way in which an electron stream is directed at a TV screen to produce an image. The stimulated light emitted from each point on the screen must be collected and converted into an electrical signal. A specially designed optical system collects the stimulated light from the phosphor and couples it to a photomultiplier tube. A special optical filter must be used in front of the photomultiplier to block the stimulating light, which is many orders of magnitude higher in intensity than the light emitted from the screen.

The photomultiplier, which has a wide dynamic range, converts the varying light intensities from the screen into varying electrical signals. These electrical signals are amplified, sampled, and passed through an analog-to-digital converter to produce binary values for the brightness of each pixel. A 12-bit system can uniquely represent a value between 0 and 4095 ($2^{12} = 4096$).

During the *read-out* process, not all of the stored energy in the screen is released. To ensure the removal of any residual latent image, the storage phosphor screen is erased while still in the image processor by flooding the entire screen with high illuminance light for a short period of time. This allows the screen to be reused for repeat exposures.

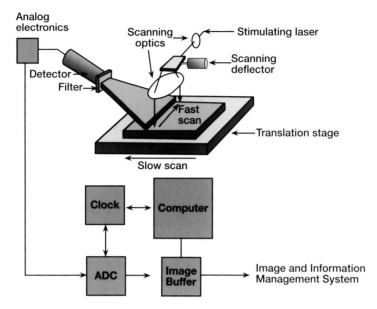

Figure 8–3 Storage Phosphor Imaging System. The latent image is stored using a storage phosphor system, and can be *read out* with a laser scanning system at a later time. A stimulating laser scans the image receptor to produce luminescence corresponding to the aerial image that exposed the image receptor. An optical detector measures the luminescence from the stimulated phosphor, producing an analog signal that is digitized and manipulated by the computer. The digital image is available for further processing by a computer or for printing using a laser printer.[18]

Storage Phosphor vs Screen-Film Imaging

Important differences between storage phosphor technology and screen-film technology in their ability to provide useful images include: latitude, dose, image quality, and noise.

Latitude

The most important difference between storage phosphor systems and screen-film systems is in *exposure latitude*. The exposure latitude of storage phosphor systems is extremely wide, about $10^4{:}1$ (10,000 times) wider than even the widest dynamic range screen-film system. As a result, storage phosphors can capture a wider range of x-ray exposure information within the aerial image than would be possible with any screen-film system. The latitude of a screen-film system is limited by the threshold ("toe") and saturation ("shoulder") portions of its characteristic curve, and also by the design compromise that must often be made between exposure latitude and film contrast.

The wide latitude of storage phosphor systems allows them to be used under a broad range of exposure conditions. The storage phosphor's latitude also makes it an ideal choice in applications where exposures are highly variable or difficult to control, for example, in portable (mobile) radiography. With appropriate digital image processing, exposures that would have required repeat exposures with a screen-film system can usually be salvaged with a storage phosphor system.

Dose
The dose requirements of a CR system depend largely upon the ability of the system to absorb and convert incident x rays into a usable signal (for example, optical density or electrical current from a photomultiplier tube). Storage phosphor systems are not inherently lower dose systems than screen-film systems. The exposure (dose) necessary to produce a reasonable image on either a screen-film system or a storage phosphor system is quite similar. In fact, some dual-screen, screen-film systems, because of their higher x-ray absorption and conversion characteristics, are somewhat more efficient in the use of x-radiation.

As the dose in any radiography system is decreased, the noise due to quantum mottle increases. As a practical matter, the lower limit on dose is determined not by any technical differences between storage phosphors and screen-film, but rather by the acceptable noise tolerance of the radiologist, who must interpret the image.

Image Quality
The image quality of any radiographic system (including storage phosphors) can be measured on an absolute scale. This absolute scale is called **detective quantum efficiency (DQE)** and it measures how efficiently a system converts input x-ray quanta into useful image signals. DQE takes into account the input and output characteristics of the system, the sharpness of the system and, especially, the input and output noise.

Storage phosphor systems have a linear, wide dynamic range compared with screen-film systems, which have a limited dynamic range (**Figure 8–4**). This characteristic also leads to a wider DQE latitude for storage phosphors. That is, storage phosphor systems have the ability to convert incoming x-ray quanta into useful output over a much wider exposure range than even the widest latitude screen-film systems. However, images made with exposures below the "useful medical range" often exhibit excessive quantum mottle. Images made with exposures above the "useful medical range" subject the patient to unnecessary radiation.

The main factor limiting sharpness (that is, the modulation transfer function, MTF) in screen-film and storage phosphor systems is virtually the same, the scattering of light within the screen. In a screen-film system, the spread of light emitted from a point in the screen (upon absorption of an x-ray quantum) spreads

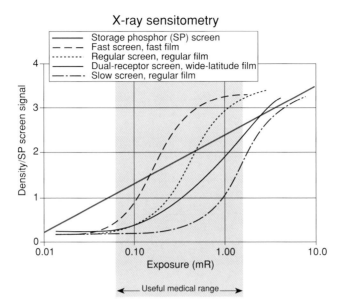

Figure 8–4 X-ray Sensitometry. The exposure requirements of storage phosphors are shown compared with a variety of screen-film combinations.

in all directions and is also scattered by other phosphor particles in the screen. By the time it reaches the interface between the screen and the film, the light spread has introduced image blur.

In storage phosphor systems, the situation is slightly different, the scatter that determines sharpness occurs with the stimulating beam rather than with the emitted light. Although the diameter of this stimulating laser beam can be quite small, the stimulating light spreads out and scatters as it passes through the depth of the screen, creating stimulated luminescence along its path. This spread of stimulated light with depth creates a blurring effect in storage phosphors similar to that resulting from the spread of emitted light in screen-film systems.

Other effects in storage phosphor systems can contribute to additional losses in sharpness. For example, sharpness is a function of the intensity of the stimulating laser light. Higher laser powers yield lower sharpness. However, higher laser powers also increase the amount of stored signal extracted from the screen. Conversely, lower laser powers increase sharpness but lower the amount of signal in the *read-out* phase. Consequently, compromises exist between laser power and image blur and signal strength in a storage phosphor system.

Another effect is the digital nature of the *read-out* process. The analog signal in the screen is spatially sampled onto a grid of points (typically about 2000 x 2000), which limits the maximum spatial frequency that the storage phosphor system can reproduce.

Noise

Storage phosphor systems have a variety of noise sources. These noise sources and their dependence on exposure and spatial frequency have a fundamental impact on the image quality limits of each system.

The most obvious source of noise is quantum mottle in the aerial image. The noise in the final image can never be lower than this inherent noise in the input x-ray beam. In fact, it will generally be greater since other noise sources contribute to the total noise of the system. Storage phosphor systems share common noise sources with screen-film systems: screen structure noise and fluctuations in the conversion and detection of x-ray photons. Additional sources of noise, peculiar to storage phosphor systems, also contribute to total image noise.

RADIOGRAPHIC DIGITIZERS

Existing analog radiographs may be scanned by a film digitizer, converting the analog optical densities of the radiograph into a series of digital pixel values in an image matrix. Once in digital matrix form, the image information can benefit from the digital image processing and management features of other digital systems.

ADVANTAGES OF DIGITAL IMAGING

Digital image data may be displayed, processed, and manipulated in a variety of ways to visualize the information in the aerial image. A 12-bit pixel can have a value from 0 to 4,095. A look-up table (LUT) is used to map the pixel values to one of the shades of gray in the displayed image (**Figure 8–5**). The digital image data may be processed to achieve image *subtraction* or *edge enhancement*. Digital image data may also be stored using magnetic or optical disks, or tape. Image data may be transferred electronically using network computer technology. The term PACS (Picture Archiving and Communication System) describes these computer-based methods of image storage and management.

One developing advantage of digital systems is in image and information management. For example, the archival storage and timely retrieval of patient images can be considerably more efficient with an electronic film library (for example, an optical disk jukebox or library) than with a traditional film library or warehouse system. The likelihood of a given image being lost or misplaced is reduced with a digital system. Furthermore, the same image (actually a digital representation of the image) can be viewed simultaneously in different locations around a hospital, facilitating easier consultation.

Digital systems also allow the transmission of images between geographically disparate locations (for example, remote primary diagnostic facilities). This ability to move images where and when they are needed makes digital systems especially attractive.

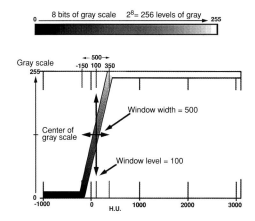

Figure 8–5 Display of Digital Images. A digital image with 12 bits per pixel can have a value from 0 to 4095. Observers cannot differentiate more than about 256 gray levels. A look-up table (LUT) is used to map each pixel value to one of the 256 shades of gray in the displayed image. The window level defines the pixel value that corresponds to the center of the gray scale. The window width defines the range of pixel values that will be shown in the range of gray shades displayed.[19]

A more immediate advantage of computed radiography and other digitizing systems is the ability to perform digital image processing. Because the acquisition and display functions in computed radiography are independent, some image processing is necessary to optimize the display of the digitized data.

The simplest form of image processing is the application of a LUT to display or print an image onto an output device. Such LUTs map the digital gray levels of the image into specific densities or luminances at the laser imager or CRT display. The particular LUT needed for a given image can depend on image source, image content, observer's preference, diagnostic application, and output device. It may be difficult to display the full acquisition dynamic range on a given output device. In this case, it is usually possible to display the image data utilizing *window width* and *window level* adjustments. The window width adjustment alters the *contrast* of the output image, while the window level alters the *brightness* of the output image.

Another form of image processing is *edge enhancement*, which usually utilizes a technique called *unsharp masking*. Unsharp masking was developed about 50 years ago by the printing industry as a photographic technique to sharpen images and to improve color reproduction. Edge enhancement lends itself very well to implementation on a computer and it has been found useful in many other applications, including medical imaging.

Subtraction

Sometimes a radiograph contains so much information that structures of diagnostic interest are obscured. For example, a lesion may be difficult to see because of the superimposed images of overlying or underlying structures. This problem frequently occurs in angiograms and may be lessened by the use of **digital subtraction**. In this technique, a digital image is selected as the mask, usually an image taken before contrast material has been injected into the patient. The value of each pixel in the mask is then subtracted from subsequent images (frame by frame). The result is a sequence of images where the background information has been largely eliminated, making even small amounts of contrast material stand out. Appendix F describes a conventional subtraction technique that does not utilize digitized image data.

Image Management

Once in digital form, electronic images may be stored and transferred by the use of a computer network. A *local area network* (LAN) allows image data to be transferred from one area of a facility to another via copper wires or fiber-optic cables. Such a system enables, for example, a hospital intensive care unit staff to retrieve images from a study performed in the radiology department, view them on a remote viewing station, and print the images using a laser printer. A *wide area network* (WAN) allows the transmission of image data between different sites via telephone, microwave or other transmission media, for example, between a large medical facility and several of its outlying clinics.

The significant advantages of these image management systems include image transfer, storage space savings, and minimal loss of images.

LASER PRINTERS

While electronic image transfer offers many advantages, the need for hard copy images is likely to continue. Hard copy of electronic digital images is accomplished by the use of a laser printer to transfer the image to film (**Figure 8–6**). Silver halide film can be made sensitive to light from the laser in the same way that x-ray film is sensitive to the blue or green light emitted by intensifying screens. Most laser films must be handled in *total* darkness because they are sensitive to the light spectrum emitted by safelights.

Laser printers provide consistent image quality and high levels of productivity for capturing images by digital modalities. In general, printers are capable of connecting to multiple imaging devices through the use of electronic interfaces that accept either video or digital image data. The image data received from each interface is stored in the printer memory. This image data, in the form of pixels

Laser printer

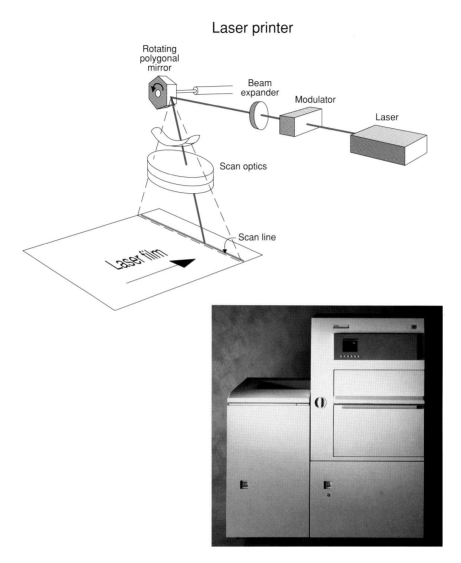

Figure 8–6 Laser Printer. Digital image data can be transferred to film using a laser printer. The output of a laser is varied to correspond to the gray scale level for each pixel using a modulator. A rotating mirror rapidly scans the beam across the width of a sheet of laser film. **(Top)** A transport system slowly moves the laser film lengthwise through the scanned laser beam to "paint" the image across the entire film. **(Bottom)** A laser printer docked to an automatic film processor.

(*pic*ture *el*ements), is represented on film in the form of gray levels. Eight-bit printers exhibit exposure modulation that provides a total of 256 gray levels, while 12-bit printers feature exposure modulation that provides a total of 4,096 gray levels. This range of gray levels helps assure continuous-tone reproduction of images without the introduction of artifacts.

All laser printers utilize interpolation, a process that increases the number of pixels to enlarge the image to the desired printed image size. Two methods of interpolation are generally used: smooth and sharp. An example of smooth interpolation is cubic spline; an example of sharp interpolation is replication. Cubic spline interpolation increases the original size of an image by calculating new pixel values from the original data. It also preserves image detail and provides a more faithful representation of the original image data than simple linear interpolation. Sharp interpolation (replication) increases the original data by repeating the original image pixel, depending on the required amount of enlargement. Differences between adjacent pixels are more noticeable in images enlarged using the sharp interpolation method.

Laser printers have dramatically increased the efficiency of radiology departments. When a laser printer docks directly to a processor, the technologist no longer must leave the patient to process films. In total roomlight operations, hard copy digital images are printed and processed in less than two minutes.

In a network environment, one or more laser printers can interface with multiple sources of digital images, providing high productivity, flexibility, and backup in producing hard copy images (**Figures 8–7** and **8–8**).

SUMMARY

All medical imaging systems use similar approaches to the three phases of the imaging cycle, which are: 1) producing the aerial image, 2) capturing and displaying the aerial image, and 3) recording and archiving the visual image.

Analog systems make use of continuously variable signals in the image capture and recording phases. Screen-film imaging is one example of an analog system. Electronic imaging systems use signals that are sampled (non-continuous) values of the imaging parameter. The sampled values are represented numerically as pixels in a digital image matrix.

Storage phosphor systems record the latent image on a screen for subsequent *read out* by specialized laser scanning systems. The result is a digital image that can be reviewed on a CRT and manipulated by a computer. These digitized images offer advantages in image processing (subtraction and edge enhancement) and image management.

Digital images from a variety of sources (imaging modalities) may be reproduced on film by a laser printer. Digital imaging networks may be used to transfer images to different locations within an institution, or between geographically remote facilities.

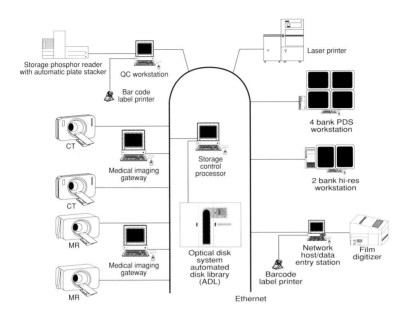

Figure 8–7 PACS Network Architecture. Digital images from multiple sources can be stored, manipulated, viewed, and printed at multiple locations by the use of a PACS network.

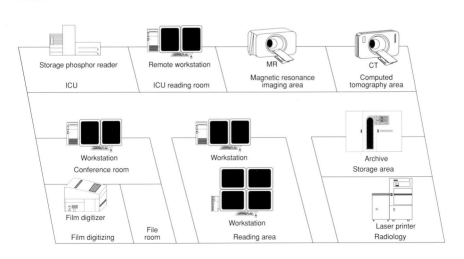

Figure 8–8 PACS Floor Plan. A typical floor plan showing the implementation of a PACS system is shown.

Calculating Changes in Exposure Factors

The most common factors that the operator can control in making an x-ray exposure are:

- milliamperage,
- exposure time,
- focal-film distance, and
- kilovoltage.

Because each of these factors makes an essential contribution to the final result, each can be altered as conditions require. In practice, changing one factor requires making an adjustment in one of the others if comparable radiographs are to be produced. Charts are available that will quickly provide the answers to these various problems. However, it is important to understand the mathematics involved so that adjustments can be handled accurately when charts are not available.

For convenience, the following symbols are used in discussing the relationships of factors involved in exposure and how they can be interchanged.

OM = original milliamperage
NM = new milliamperage
OT = original time
NT = new time
OD = original distance
ND = new distance
OmAs = original milliampere-seconds
NmAs = new milliampere-seconds

MILLIAMPERAGE-TIME RELATIONSHIP

The milliamperage (mA) required for a given exposure is inversely proportional to the exposure time. That is, the shorter the exposure time, the higher the mA; and the longer the exposure time, the lower the mA for that exposure. This rule can be expressed by the following equation:

$$\frac{\text{original milliamperage}}{\text{new milliamperage}} = \frac{\text{new time}}{\text{original time}}$$

or by using the symbols

$$\frac{\text{OM}}{\text{NM}} = \frac{\text{NT}}{\text{OT}}$$

This formula may be solved for either new factor,

$$NT = \frac{(OM)(OT)}{NM} \quad \text{or} \quad NM = \frac{(OM)(OT)}{NT}$$

Problem 1: A milliamperage (OM) of 50 and an exposure time (OT) of 1/2 (0.5) second have been used. To stop motion, it is necessary to decrease the exposure time (NT) to 1/20 (0.05) second. What mA (NM) would be required?

Solution 1: As we have seen above, the new mA is equal to the original mA multiplied by the original time, divided by the new time. Thus:

$$NM = \frac{(OM)(OT)}{NT}$$

Substituting the known values, we have:

$$NT = \frac{(50)(0.5)}{0.05} = \frac{25}{0.05} = 500 \text{ mA}$$

Problem 2: Suppose that 50 mA (OM) and an exposure time (OT) of 2 seconds have been used, and you want to increase the mA (NM) to 100. What exposure time (NT) would be required?

Solution 2: Using the formula, and solving for NT, we have:

$$NT = \frac{(OM)(OT)}{NM} = \frac{(50)(2)}{100} = 1 \text{ second}$$

Milliampere Seconds

The unit for the product of milliamperage and time is **milliampere seconds** (**mAs**), and it can be considered as the single factor that controls the quantity of exposure if the kilovoltage remains fixed.

FOCAL-FILM DISTANCE RELATIONSHIP

Inverse Square Law

X rays that are not scattered diverge along straight paths and cover an increasingly larger area with diminishing x-ray fluence as they travel from their source. The relationship between distance and x-ray fluence is called the **inverse**

square law, because the *fluence* of the radiation varies inversely as the *square* of the distance from the source of radiation (focal spot).

Changes in Focal-Film Distance

Three major reasons exist for changing focal-film distance.

1. Geometric blurring, magnification, and distortion are reduced by an increase in focal-film distance (assuming no change in object-film distance). However, this increase in distance is limited in practice by the capacity of the tube, since an increase in focal-film distance requires an increase in the quantity of x rays generated if the same optical density is to be maintained in the radiograph.

2. When a Potter-Bucky diaphragm (grid) is used, the tube should be operated at the distance for which the grid is designed, usually 40 inches [100 cm]. The higher the *grid ratio,* the less margin available in selecting the focal-film distance. For example, a grid with a 5:1 ratio generally allows focal-film distances ranging from about 28 [71 cm] to 72 inches [180 cm]. A grid with a 16:1 ratio usually has a fixed focal-film distance, typically 40 inches [100 cm] (**Figure 3-8**).

3. Splints, casts or other appliances may prevent optimum positioning of the patient and may require a change from a usual focal-film distance. This most commonly occurs during radiography performed at the bedside.

To obtain proper film densities, *inverse square law* corrections must be applied (**Figure 2–14**).

TIME-DISTANCE RELATIONSHIP

When focal-film distance is changed, the total amount of x-ray fluence must be increased or decreased in order to make a comparable exposure using the new distance (ND). This can be done by changing the mA that governs the rate at which the tube produces x-radiation, or by adjusting exposure time.

If the original exposure time (OT) required for a given exposure and the original distance (OD) are known, the new exposure time (NT) for any new distance (ND) can be calculated. The *inverse square law* states that the fluence of the x-ray beam varies inversely as the square of the distance from the source (focal spot). To produce a given optical density at a different distance, therefore, it is necessary to vary the exposure directly as the square of the distance. This means that the exposure must be increased for an increase in distance or decreased for a decrease in distance.

The formula for time-distance relationships is:

$$\frac{\text{New time}}{\text{Original time}} = \frac{(\text{New distance})^2}{(\text{Original distance})^2}$$

or in symbols

$$\frac{NT}{OT} = \frac{(ND)^2}{(OD)^2}$$

Problem 1: Suppose that the original exposure time (OT) is 2 seconds, and the original distance (OD) is 100 centimeters. What time (NT) would be required if the distance (ND) is reduced to 75 centimeters?

Solution 1: From the original formula, solving for the new time (NT)

$$NT = \frac{(OT)\,(ND)^2}{(OD)^2}$$

and substituting numerical values in this formula gives

$$NT = \frac{(2)\,(75)^2}{(100)^2} = \frac{(2)\,(5625)}{10,000} = 1.125 \text{ seconds}$$

Problem 2: Suppose that the original exposure time (OT) is 1/2 second and the distance (OD) is 72 inches. It is desired to decrease the exposure time (NT) to 1/10 (0.1) second. What new distance (ND) will be required?

Solution 2: From the original formula, solving for the new distance $(ND)^2$

$$(ND)^2 = \frac{(NT)\,(OD)^2}{OT}$$

and substituting numerical values in this formula gives

$$(ND)^2 = \frac{(0.1)\,(72)^2}{0.5} = \frac{(0.1)\,(5184)}{0.5} = \frac{(518.4)}{0.5} = 1036.8$$

Solving for ND, we find by taking the square root,

$$ND = \sqrt{1036.8} = 32 \text{ inches, approximately.}$$

MILLIAMPERAGE-DISTANCE RELATIONSHIP

The arithmetic involved in solving problems of milliamperage-distance relationships is essentially the same as for time-distance relationships because mA and time affect exposure in the same way.

The general formula for the milliamperage-distance relationship is

$$\frac{NM}{OM} = \frac{(ND)^2}{(OD)^2}$$

MILLIAMPERE-SECONDS AND DISTANCE RELATIONSHIP

The product of mA and time is commonly considered as a single factor. The most useful calculations involving distance are those that combine these two factors into one, **milliampere-seconds (mAs)**. The original mAs value is represented by *OmAs*, the new value by *NmAs*.

The mAs and distance formula is expressed

$$\frac{\text{New mAs}}{\text{Original mAs}} = \frac{(\text{New Distance})^2}{(\text{Original Distance})^2}$$

or

$$\frac{NmAs}{OmAs} = \frac{(ND)^2}{(OD)^2}$$

Problem 1: Suppose that 100 mAs (OmAs) are required for an exposure at a distance (OD) of 72 inches. What distance (ND) will be required to permit the reduction of the mAs (NmAs) to 25?

Solution 1: Solving the formula for $(ND)^2$ we have the equation:

$$(ND)^2 = \frac{(NmAs)\,(OD)^2}{OmAs}$$

$$ND^2 = \frac{(25)\,(72)^2}{(100)} = \frac{(25)\,(5184)}{100} = 1296$$

Then, $ND = \sqrt{1296} = 36$ inches

Problem 2: Suppose that the usual factors for a radiograph of the pelvis are a distance (OD) of 100 centimeters and 100 mAs (OmAs). The patient cannot be moved to the table, and the bed height permits a maximum distance (ND) of only 88 centimeters. What new mAs (NmAs) value will be required?

Solution 2: The formula is

$$NmAs \quad = \quad \frac{(OmAs) \ (ND)^2}{(OD)^2}$$

Substituting the known values, we have:

$$NmAs \quad = \quad \frac{(100) \ (88)^2}{(100)^2} \quad = \quad \frac{(100) \ (7744)}{10,000} \quad = \quad 77.4 \ mAs$$

KILOVOLTAGE CHANGES

Conditions often arise that require a change in kilovoltage (kVp). This necessitates a compensating change in mAs or distance. However, an increase in kilovoltage, with the exposure adjusted to maintain the same average density, will produce lower contrast in the radiograph because x rays generated at a higher kVp reduce subject contrast. Conversely, a decrease in kVp will produce higher contrast.

The relationship between kVp and exposure is complex. When kVp is raised, all energies present in the lower kVp beam are present in the higher kVp beam and in greater numbers, along with new, higher energies not previously present.

The effect of kVp changes on the beam fluence reaching the image receptor depends on such factors as type of examination, patient size and age, as well as the type of x-ray machine used.

AUTOMATIC EXPOSURE CONTROL

There was a time when kVp, mA, time, and distance had to be decided upon and set manually for each radiographic exposure. Today, however, electronic devices are often used to select radiographic exposure factors. The first devices of this type were designed to control exposure time. They fall into two categories: **phototimers** and **ionization chambers.**

Phototimers

Phototimers contain a fluorescent material that emits light when exposed to the x-ray beam. The light is directed toward a photocathode that emits electrons when struck by light. The number of electrons emitted is proportional to the brightness of the light, which in turn is proportional to the x-ray fluence striking the fluorescent screen. This flow of electrons is amplified in a *photomultiplier* and, after passing through appropriate circuits, automatically terminates the exposure when a predetermined radiation level has been reached.

The phototimer is often located behind the cassette to avoid casting a shadow on the radiograph. For this reason, cassettes that contain thin lead backing or no lead backing are used with phototimed machines so that sufficient x-ray fluence reaches the phototimer to provide satisfactory exposure control.

Ionization Chambers

Ionization chambers contain two thin, flat radiolucent electrodes with air between them. When placed in an x-ray beam, the air between the electrodes is ionized, that is, charged particles or ions are formed. If a voltage is applied across the electrodes, the ions are attracted to them causing a current to flow. This current is proportional to the fluence of the x-ray beam. When amplified and measured through auxiliary circuits, this current may be used to automatically stop the production of x rays when the correct exposure has been delivered. Because of their low x-ray absorption, ionization chambers, if large enough, can be located between the patient and the cassette without casting any interfering shadows onto the radiograph.

It is customary to locate two or three of these ionization chambers or exposure detectors in the irradiated field to sample x-ray fluences in various locations, and to average their combined effect. Operating controls are provided to permit selection of the ionization chamber or phototimer combination best suited to monitor a particular examination.

Programmed Exposures

With the ready availability of microcomputers, controls now exist for x-ray machines that automatically select kVp, mA, and exposure time. A press of a button designates the examination to be performed and allows for differences in patient absorption. Most units also provide the option to switch to full manual control.

In spite of the advent of such automatically controlled equipment, it is still important to learn the relationships discussed in this appendix. An understanding of the principles involved and the ability to apply them is the key to obtaining high-quality radiographs. Automatic equipment can malfunction, and the knowledgeable person is in a much better position to detect errors and to correct them.

Metric Units and Conversion Factors

This appendix contains some of the units, symbols, prefixes, and conversion factors used in the International System of Units (SI).

UNITS, SYMBOLS, AND PREFIXES

Base Units

Quantity	Unit	Symbol
length	meter	m
mass	kilogram	kg
time	second	s
electric current	ampere	A
thermodynamic temperature	kelvin	K
amount of substance	mole	mol
luminous intensity	candela	cd
power	watt	W
force	newton	N

Derived Units

Quantity	Unit	Symbol	Definition
absorbed dose	gray	Gy	J/kg
activity (of radionuclides)	becquerel	Bq	(disintegrations)/s
area	square meter	m^2	
density (mass density)	kilogram per cubic meter	kg/m^3	
electric charge, quantity of electricity	coulomb	C	A·s
electrical potential, electromotive force, potential difference	volt	V	W/A
energy, work quantity of heat	joule	J	N·m
frequency	hertz	Hz	(cycle)/s

Units in Use with SI

Quantity	Unit	Symbol	Definition
time	minute	min	1 min = 60 s
	hour	h	1 h = 60 min
			= 3,600 s
	day	d	1 d = 24 h
			= 86,400 s
temperature	degree Celsius	°C	
volume (fluid)	liter	L	1 L = 10^{-3} m^3
activity (for radionuclides)	curie	Ci	1 Ci = 3.7 x 10^{10}Bq
exposure	roentgen	R	1 R = 2.58 x 10^{-4}C/kg
absorbed dose	rad	rd	1 rd = 0.01 Gy

SI Prefixes

Factors by Which the Unit is Multiplied		Prefix	Symbol
1 000 000 000 000 000 000	= 10^{18}	exa	E
1 000 000 000 000 000	= 10^{15}	peta	P
1 000 000 000 000	= 10^{12}	tera	T
1 000 000 000	= 10^{9}	giga	G
1 000 000	= 10^{6}	mega	M
1 000	= 10^{3}	kilo	k
100	= 10^{2}	hecto	h
10	= 10	deka	da
0.1	= 10^{-1}	deci	d
0.01	= 10^{-2}	centi	c
0.001	= 10^{-3}	milli	m
0.000 001	= 10^{-6}	micro	μ
0.000 000 001	= 10^{-9}	nano	n
0.000 000 000 001	= 10^{-12}	pico	p
0.000 000 000 000 001	= 10^{-15}	femto	f
0.000 000 000 000 000 001	= 10^{-18}	atto	a

Examples:

1,000 volts	=	1 kilovolt	=	1 kV
0.01 meter	=	1 centimeter	=	1 cm
1,000,000 hertz	=	1 megahertz	=	1 MHz
0.000 001 second	=	1 microsecond	=	1 μs
0.000 000 546 meter	=	546 nanometers	=	546 nm

CONVERSION FACTORS

Length or distance

1 inch = 25.4 mm = 2.54 cm
1 foot = 30.5 cm
1 yard = 0.914 m
1 mile = 1.6 km

1 meter = 39.4 inches (in.) = 3.28 feet (ft) = 1.09 yards (yd)
1 kilometer = 0.62 mile

Volume (fluid)

1.0 milliliter (mL)	=	1 cubic centimeter
	=	3.38×10^{-2} fluidounces (fl oz)
	=	6.10×10^{-2} cubic inches (in.^{3})
1 quart (US)	=	0.95 liter (L)
1 gallon (US)	=	3.79 liters (L)

Mass

1 ounce   =   28.4 grams
1 pound   =   454 grams
1 kilogram   =   2.2 pounds (lb)   =   35.3 ounces (oz)

Temperature

To convert degrees Fahrenheit to degrees Celsius, subtract 32 from the Fahrenheit temperature and divide by 1.8. Conversely, to convert degrees Celsius to degrees Fahrenheit, multiply the Celsius temperature by 1.8 and add 32.

Examples

F	C	
0	-17.8	
14	-10	
32	0	Freezing point for water
50	10	
60	15.6	
68	20	Typical room temperature
77	25	
90	32.2	
98.6	37	Normal body temperature
100	37.8	
212	100	Boiling point for water

Fourier Transform and Modulation Transfer Function (MTF)

FOURIER THEORY

The Fourier theory asserts that any waveform can be reconstructed as the weighted sum of sine and cosine curves. The lowest frequency present is called the *fundamental*. The additional weighted sines and cosines required to reconstruct the waveform are even multiples of the fundamental frequency, called *harmonics*. This theorem will ultimately be applied to the line spread function, but first consider its application to a more familiar subject, music.

You are probably aware that a band or orchestra often plays music that has been written out using musical notation. The group tunes their instruments so that no instrument is either sharp or flat, which would produce a discordant sound. In the United States, instruments are tuned based on a sound frequency of 440 Hz, which corresponds to a pitch we call *concert A*. Since each musician tunes his or her instrument to the same note, how is it possible that we can distinguish among the concert A pitch played by a violin, a flute or a saxophone? The answer brings us closer to an understanding of the Fourier theory.

When each of the instruments plays the concert A pitch, each produces a complex sound wave that is not a pure sine wave, but has a common fundamental frequency of 440 Hz. This common fundamental frequency is the reason that we describe the note as an A. The unique sound of the long tones played by each instrument is determined by the harmonics, or overtones, produced by each instrument (**Figure C–1**). When properly trained, our ears can recognize both the common fundamental frequency and the different harmonics, allowing us to distinguish the sounds of different instruments.

An electronic music synthesizer is a common instrument in many jazz and pop orchestras. A music synthesizer is usually a keyboard-type instrument that is capable of producing sounds that imitate a number of other instruments, such as violins, flutes and saxophones, as well as creating unique new electronic synthesized sounds. A synthesizer contains many electronic sine wave generators. When the musician plays a concert A pitch on the keyboard, the synthesizer sets the fundamental frequency at 440 Hz, as well as even multiples of the fundamental frequency (880, 1320, 1760 Hz). When the flute sound is selected, the synthesizer creates these sounds by selecting the weighting factors (relative volumes) of the harmonics that correspond to the Fourier transform of the tones produced by a real flute. The result is a very realistic sounding synthesized flute sound. In order to change from a flute sound to a saxophone sound, the musician makes a selection that changes the weighting factors of the harmonics to correspond to the sound of a sax, and so on.

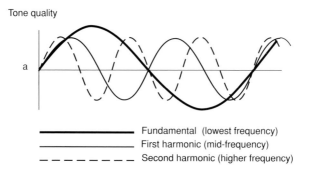

Tone quality

a

——————————— Fundamental (lowest frequency)
——————————— First harmonic (mid-frequency)
– – – – – – – – – Second harmonic (higher frequency)

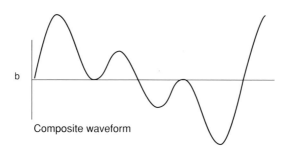

b

Composite waveform

Figure C–1 The Application of the Fourier Theory in Music. The Fourier Theory states that a complex sound wave may be reproduced as the sum of sine and cosine waves. For a *concert A* pitch, the fundamental frequency is 440 Hz. **(a)** The first harmonic is 880 Hz; the second harmonic is 1320 Hz. **(b)** The complex wave produced by a violin may be synthesized with a weighted sum of the fundamental frequency and higher harmonic frequencies.

The use of the Fourier theory to synthesize different sounds is not a new idea. The same basic concepts have been used for centuries to control the way in which pipe organs alter the tonal quality of the many sounds they can produce.

Audio frequency is another familiar musical concept that can be applied to the discussion of image quality. Anyone who has ever used a home or car hi-fi system has experimented with the bass and treble controls found on such equipment. When the bass is boosted, the volume of *low-frequency* sounds in the music, such as an electric bass or bass drum, is increased. *High-frequency* sounds, such as flutes and cymbals, are increased in volume when the treble setting is increased. Compare the sound waveforms for a low-frequency sine wave (the fundamental) and a high-frequency sine wave (the upper harmonics) in **Figure C–1**. It is clear that a high-frequency wave changes from its lowest to its highest value in much less time than does a low-frequency sound wave.

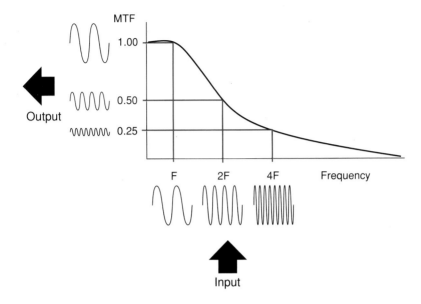

Figure C–2 Spatial Frequencies and the Modulation Transfer Function (MTF). This MTF describes the ability of an imaging system to reproduce low (F), medium (2F), and high (4F) spatial frequency information. Note that the height (amplitude) of the three input spatial frequencies is equal because the MTF value is 1.00 at frequency F and the output wave is equal in height to the input wave. As the MTF values decrease for higher frequencies, so does the height of the output waves.

The concept of **spatial frequency** used in imaging may be more easily understood by analogy with the more familiar concept of audio frequency. Spatial frequency is measured in units of cycles per mm, while audio frequency is measured in cycles per second. Audio frequency is a rate of change of sound pressure with respect to time (Hz or cycles/second), while *spatial frequency is a rate of change of optical density with respect to distance or space (line pairs per millimeter)*. In a radiograph, low spatial frequencies correspond to gradual changes in optical density with distance, similar to low audio frequencies changing gradually in sound pressure with time. *Portions of an image where optical densities change from high to low values over a short distance are said to contain high spatial frequency information*. In **Figure C–2**, the modulation transfer function (MTF) describes the ability of an imaging system to reproduce low (F), medium (2F), and high (4F) spatial frequency information.

In medical imaging, both low and high spatial frequencies are clinically important. Low spatial frequency image components provide useful diagnostic information when examining an image of the abdomen, where gradual changes in optical densities in some anatomical regions may indicate the presence of pathology. The high spatial frequency information contained in an extremity radiograph or mammogram indicates fine detail and structure within these organs. Medical radiographic images contain the full range of low, medium, and high spatial frequency information.

MODULATION TRANSFER FUNCTION

Recall the slit assembly used in **Figure 7–7** to produce the line spread function in **Figure 7–8**. If the imaging system were perfect, the line spread function would be a rectangle, with perfectly vertical sides and a width equal to that of the slit. Because the rise of the curve is infinitely steep (a vertical line has infinite slope), the perfect image of the slit contains infinitely high frequency information. In fact, such a slit image contains all possible frequencies of information.

An imaging system must have a perfect 100% response at all spatial frequencies in order for the line spread function to be a perfect rectangle, that is, the image would have to be a perfect rendition of the object. If the image exhibits a loss of about one-half of the information, the response value is 50%. If the response of this perfect system were plotted on a scale of 0 to 100%, one would see the upper most horizontal straight line in **Figure 7–8**.

However, real-world imaging systems are imperfect; their frequency responses fall off rapidly from 100% as spatial frequency is increased. **Figure 7–8** shows the frequency response, or modulation transfer function, derived by calculating the Fourier transform of the line spread function.

It is important to distinguish between the line spread function and modulation transfer function curves because their similar general shape can lead to confusion. The x-axis for the line spread function is in units of length, usually in micrometers or millimeters, while the x-axis for a modulation transfer function is in units of spatial frequency, usually in cycles per mm, or mm[-1]. When comparing imaging systems, the line spread function of a higher blur system will be *wider* than a sharper system, as seen with Film A in **Figure 7–8**. However, the modulation transfer function of a sharper system is closer to the ideal case (Film B in **Figure 7–8**) and therefore is above the modulation transfer function for an imaging system with greater blur (Film A in **Figure 7–8**).

The total blur in an imaging system is a combination of the blur introduced by the focal spot size (geometric blur), image receptor (screen blur), and motion. Modulation transfer functions may be determined for each factor separately. Since each value on a modulation transfer function curve is between 0 and 100%, the *system MTF* (the combined effect of each component) may be determined by multiplying together the MTFs of all components. Some MTF curves are plotted on a 0 to 1.0 y-axis scale, which is equivalent to the 0 to 100% scale shown in **Figure 7–8**. The MTF of the entire system will always be below the curves of each contributing component (**Figure C–3**).

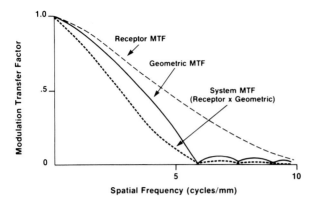

Figure C–3 System Modulation Transfer Function (MTF). Curves for the MTFs associated with geometric and receptor blur are shown. The system MTF is calculated by multiplying (at each frequency) the geometric and receptor MTFs. Note that the system MTF curve will always lie below MTFs of individual components of the system.[15]

Troubleshooting Processor Performance and Artifacts

MONITORING FILM PROCESSOR PERFORMANCE

The following charts identify the major causes and remedies for unwanted increases and decreases in speed, contrast, and fog.

Speed and Contrast Suddenly Increasing

Cause	Remedy
High developer temperature*	(a) Check the developer temperature. (b) Check that the water temperature in the wash tank is not too high; it should be 5°F (3°C) below the normal working temperature of the developer. (Not applicable in the case of processors in which the developer temperature is controlled independently of the water temperature; consult the processor operating manual.) (c) Adjust the water temperature, if necessary, and wait for the developer temperature to drop. (d) If the water temperature is correct but the developer temperature is high, adjust the developer temperature control and allow for the developer temperature to drop.
Slow processor transport speed	Check the transport of the processor and correct the speed if necessary. (Consult the processor operating manual.)

Speed and Contrast Gradually Increasing Over a Period of Time

Cause	Remedy
Overreplenishment of the developer	(a) Check to see if the total amount of film being processed has changed. If it has, adjust the replenishment rates to match the new conditions and the predominant film size being used. (b) If the total amount of film being processed has not changed, check the replenishment rates and adjust them if necessary.
Fixer exhausted	(a) Check the silver content of the fixer solution in the tank by using silver estimating papers. The silver content should not exceed 10 g/liter. (b) Check the fixer replenishment rate and adjust it if necessary.

*A temperature increase of up to 4°F (2°C) is assumed here. Much larger increases may lead to an increase in fog, sufficient to result in a net *reduction* in contrast.

Speed and Contrast Suddenly Decreasing

Cause	Remedy
Low developer temperature	(a) Check the developer temperature. (b) Check that the water temperature in the wash tank is not too low; it should be 5°F (3°C) below the normal working temperature of the developer. (Note: in processors where the developer temperature is controlled independently of the water temperature, the 5°F (3°C) does not apply. For these processors, consult the processor operating manual to determine the correct water temperature in the wash tank.) (c) If necessary, adjust the water temperature and wait for the developer temperature to rise. (d) If the water temperature is correct but the developer temperature is low, adjust the temperature control and allow for the developer temperature to rise.
Poor recirculation	Check that recirculation is taking place; if it is not, consult your local service specialist.
Fast processor transport speed	Check the transport speed of the processor and correct it if necessary. (Consult the processor operating manual.)

Speed and Contrast Gradually Decreasing Over a Period of Time

Cause	Remedy
Underreplenishment of the developer	(a) Check to see if the total amount of film being processed has changed. If it has, adjust the replenishment rates to match the new conditions and the predominant film size being used. (b) If the total amount of film being processed has not changed, check the replenishment rates and adjust them if necessary.

Speed and Fog Rapidly Increasing, While the Contrast is Decreasing

Cause	Remedy
Developer contaminated with fixer	Change the developer solution and determine what caused the contamination. Then eliminate the cause of the contamination.
Faulty safelights	(a) Turn all the safelights off and process another control strip. If the new strip is still fogged, safelights are not the cause. (b) If the safelights are at fault: (1) check their filters for cracks or fading, (2) ensure that the correct wattage lamp is installed in the safelights, and (3) check that the safelights are the correct distance from the workbench.
Control strips fogged (but there have been no density changes in the clinical films)	Process an additional control strip. If the new strip is fogged, replace the existing box of QC film with a new box, and expose a new set of strips.

FILM PROCESSING ARTIFACTS

Artifacts may result from processing, handling, equipment, and grids. The following chart describes common processing artifacts, their causes, and suggested corrective actions.

Processing Artifact Identification Chart

Artifact	Possible cause	Correction
Artifacts that run parallel to the direction of film travel		
(1) Processor guide shoe marks		
Generally 2.5 cm (1 in.) apart; they may appear as a plus or a minus density	A bent, loose or dirty processor guide shoe	Inspect guide shoes and correct problem conditions
The marks may extend the full length of the film or they may appear intermittently	A problem with rollers or bearings in one of the processor rack "turnarounds"	Tighten or replace the guide shoe, if necessary, the guide shoe mounting bracket
Note: shoe marks up to 6.4 mm (1/4 in.) long on the leading and trailing edge of the film are considered acceptable		Inspect and replace bearings and rollers as necessary
(2) Surface drying streaks		
These appear on the surface of the film as slight variations in density	A problem with the amount of spring pressure on the wash rack squeegee rollers, or dirty squeegee rollers	Inspect and replace squeegee roller springs as necessary
		Clean the wash rack squeegee rollers
	The dryer temperature is too high, or the dryer air tube(s) are out of position	Check the position of dryer air tubes
		Use the lowest dryer temperature that will adequately dry the films
(3) Delay streaks		
Uneven plus and minus density lines on the leading edge of the film	Excessive time has elapsed since feeding the film into the processor	Feed a clean-up film if the processor has been inoperative for an extended period
	The processor has been improperly vented	Correct ventilation problems. Consult the processor manufacturer's recommendations

Processing Artifact Identification Chart

Artifact	Possible cause	Correction
Artifacts that run perpendicular to the direction of film travel		
(4) Hesitation lines		
Plus density lines running across the film. The lines may be evenly or unevenly spaced	Film hesitation is primarily caused by a problem in the developer processing rack	Inspect and repair the developer processing rack. Inspect the developer rack "turnaround" section for loose or broken parts
	Exhausted or underreplenished developer solution	Check that the replenishment system is operating correctly, and that the replenishment rates are adjusted according to the film manufacturer's recommendations
Random direction		
(5) Static marks		
A plus density artifact that may appear randomly across the film as small well-defined spots or may resemble a tree branch	Low humidity, poor grounding of the processor and film handling equipment, or careless handling of film by the operator	Operate the processor within recommended temperature and humidity levels
		Ground the processing and film handling equipment properly
		Instruct operators on proper film handling techniques
(6) Flame pattern		
Density variations on a film that resemble a flame pattern	Usually caused by a too high or too low recirculation rate	Check that the developer filter is changed regularly according to the processor manufacturer's recommendations
		Only the processor manufacturer's recommended orifice should be installed in the developer recirculation system

Processing Artifact Identification Chart

Artifact	Possible cause	Correction
Random direction		
(7) Run back		
Occurs on the trailing edge of the film and has the appearance of wavy plus and minus density areas on the film	Caused by incomplete removal of developer as the film is entering the fixer solution. This allows the developer to run down the film, creating variations in film density	Clean the processor cross-over assemblies daily in warm water To minimize this problem, roller modifications are available for some processors
(8) Wet pressure		
Overall blotchy or grainy appearance of the film	Buildup on rollers in developer rack	Clean the processor regularly
	Use of abrasive cleaning materials on processing rack rollers	Use non-abrasive cleaning materials
	Improper chemical replenishment rates	Adjust replenishment rates according to the film manufacturer's recommendations

Manual Method of Time-Temperature Processing

Time-temperature processing of radiographic film is an effective means of converting the invisible latent image into a diagnostically useful radiograph. This technique is important at facilities that are without automatic processing capabilities, even temporarily.

X-ray processing solutions are most effective when used within a comparatively narrow range of temperatures. At temperatures below those recommended, some of the chemicals are definitely sluggish in action, which may cause underdevelopment and inadequate fixation. At temperatures much above those recommended, activity is too high for manual processing control. Such high temperatures may soften the emulsion to such an extent that it is easily damaged. In fact, processing temperatures should not be above the film manufacturer's recommendations.

The processing temperatures prescribed by the film manufacturer are generally recommended for several reasons. First, good sensitometric performance of the film is obtained; that is, the contrast and speed of the film are satisfactory and fog is kept to an acceptably low level. Second, the processing time is practical; and third, with modern solution heating and cooling, the temperature is usually conveniently maintained.

For these reasons, every effort should be made to keep the solutions at the recommended temperature during use. By doing so, the user can obtain the best sensitometric characteristics and will also have the advantage of a standardized time of development, fixation, and washing.

Whenever it is necessary to work with solutions at other than the recommended temperature but within a range acceptable to the film manufacturer, an adjustment must be made in processing procedure. This adjustment consists of increasing or decreasing the time of development (depending on the temperature), and ensuring adequate fixation in a relatively fresh solution. *As developer temperature increases, development time decreases and vice versa.* This procedure of adjusting time to suit the temperature is known as **time-temperature processing**.

Time-temperature processing is preferable to processing by visual inspection, which actually requires more attention and demands greater skill and judgment. Variations in eye accommodation, the low level of illumination in the darkroom, and the opacity of the uncleared film, all make processing by inspection difficult and subject to error. Such "sight development" should be avoided. When time and temperature are carefully correlated, as recommended by the film manufacturer, any lack of density in the radiographs can be attributed to underexposure, not to underdevelopment; and excessive density can be charged to overexposure rather than to overdevelopment. This is important in determining adjustments in exposure. Problems have been detected where excessive radiation exposure has been combined with underdeveloping to produce an image that appeared acceptable using sight development. The increased patient dose and loss of image quality from this error in technique can be avoided by using a constant time-temperature method.

REPLENISHMENT FOR MANUAL DEVELOPMENT

The activity of an underreplenished developer gradually diminishes by exhaustion; that is, as it is used, its developing power decreases, partly because of the consumption of the developing agent in changing the exposed silver halide to metallic silver, and partly because of the restraining effect of the accumulated reaction products on the development process. The extent of this decrease in activity will depend on the number of films processed and their average density. Even when the developer is not used, the activity may decrease slowly because of aerial oxidation of the developing agent. This exhaustion, unless counteracted, will gradually result in underdevelopment and affect contrast and speed adversely. In addition, some of the developer is physically carried out of the tank with each film. These conditions must be offset in some way if uniform radiographic results are to be obtained. The best way to compensate for these losses is to use a replenisher system in which the activity and volume of the solution are maintained by suitable chemical replenishment.

A replenisher system is efficient and simple, it merely requires adding a solution to the original developer to compensate for loss of activity, thereby permitting a constant developing time. The replenisher performs the double function of maintaining both the liquid level in the tank and the activity of the solution.

With this method, films should be removed from the developer quickly to minimize the amount of excess developer that can drain back into the tank. Normally, this will carry out the proper amount of solution to permit correct replenishment. The level of the developer in the tank should be kept at a fairly constant point, the amount lost being restored by adding replenisher. After a little experience, withdrawing the correct amount of solution on the film will become automatic. When too much of the used developer remains, however, it can be removed to allow the correct amount of replenisher to be added. Replenisher should be added in amounts and at intervals recommended by the film manufacturer. Adding replenisher in relatively small quantities and stirring immediately after each addition reduces fluctuations in solution activity.

It is not practical to continue replenishment indefinitely. The best results will be obtained if the instructions given for the various types of developer are followed. In any case, the developer solution should be discarded at the end of three months because of air oxidation, accumulation of gelatin, sludge, and impurities that find their way into the solution.

PROCEDURE

Some films that have been designed for automatic processing are not suitable for manual processing and should be manually processed only in an emergency. With respect to the procedures followed in manual processing, consult the film manufacturer's recommendations, as these vary from product to product. Personnel performing the manual processing procedure should follow all manufacturers' safety recommendations. Processing sites must also be in compliance with all applicable local, state, and federal regulations regarding the introduction of waste material into the environment.

For the following procedure, see **Figure E-1**. First, using separate paddles, stir the solutions thoroughly to equalize the temperature and chemical activity throughout each tank. Next, determine solution temperatures. To avoid contamination, rinse the thermometer after contact with each solution. Set the timer for the recommended period of development based on the temperature of the developer solution. Attach the film carefully to the correct size hanger. Start the timer and immediately immerse the film in the developer. Tap the hanger against the side of the tank to remove air bubbles from the film surface. If the film manufacturer recommends agitation, follow instructions as to how frequently and vigorously to agitate. When the timer rings, remove the film hanger immediately and drain the film for a moment into the space between the tanks.

RINSING

After a film has been developed, it should be immersed in a rinse bath of clean, circulating water, or better still, a stop bath solution and, unless otherwise recommended, agitated continuously. The minimum rinsing or *stop bath time* is usually about 30 seconds. Temperatures of all solutions in the processing cycle, including the rinse bath, should be maintained within a few degrees of each other. After rinsing, the film should again be well-drained so that the least possible amount of liquid is transferred to the fixer.

FIXATION

As in the case of the developer solution, the activity of the fixer is influenced by its freshness and temperature. If the fixer solution is allowed to become warmer than recommended, abnormal emulsion swelling and slow drying of the film may occur.

Fixation should be properly timed. Films must not be taken out before fixation is completed, nor left in for prolonged periods. The total fixing time for a film should be about *twice* the clearing time, which is the time required for the complete disappearance of the original milky opaqueness of the film. It is during this time that the fixer is dissolving the undeveloped silver halide. However, an

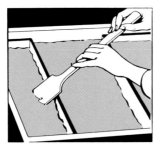

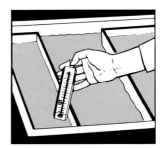

1 Stir Solutions Stir developer and fixer solutions to equalize their temperature. (Use separate paddle for each to avoid possible contamination.)

2 Check Temperature Check temperature of solutions with accurate thermometer. Rinse thermometer after each measurement to avoid contaminating next solution. Adjust to recommended temperature.

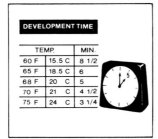

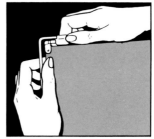

DEVELOPMENT TIME		
TEMP.		MIN.
60 F	15.5 C	8 1/2
65 F	18.5 C	6
68 F	20 C	5
70 F	21 C	4 1/2
75 F	24 C	3 1/4

3 Set Timer Set timer for recommended period of development based on temperature of developer solution.

4 Load Film on Hanger Attach film carefully to correct size hanger. (Attach at lower corners first.) Avoid finger marks, scratches, or bending.

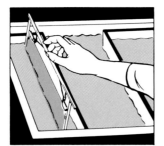

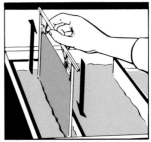

5 Immerse Film in Developer Start timer. Completely immerse film into the developer. Do it smoothly and without pause to avoid streaking. Rap film against side of tank to remove film surface air bubbles.

6 Agitate Film, If Recommended Follow the film manufacturer's instructions as to vigor and frequency and whether the film should be agitated within the tank or raised and lowered.

Figure E-1 Basic Steps for Manual Processing of X-ray Film

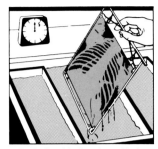

7 Drain Outside Developer Tank
When timer rings, lift hanger out immediately. Then drain film for a moment into space between tanks. For fast drainage, tilt hanger.

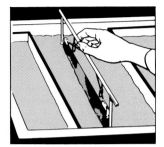

8 Rinse Thoroughly Place film in acid rinse bath or running water. Agitate hanger continuously. Rinse film about 30 seconds. Lift from rinse bath. Drain well.

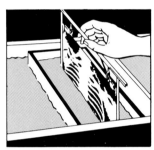

9 Fix Adequately Immerse film. Agitate hanger vigorously at start. Follow the film manufacturer's recommendations for time and temperature—at least twice the time required to "clear" film (when its milky look has disappeared).

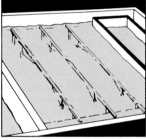

10 Wash Completely Remove film to tank of running water (flow rate of about 8 complete changes per hour). Keep ample space between hangers (water must flow over their tops). Allow adequate time for thorough washing—usually from 5 to 30 minutes, depending on film.

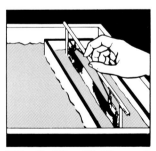

11 Use Final Rinse If facilities permit, use a final rinse in a solution containing a wetting agent to speed drying and prevent water marks. Immerse film for 30 seconds, and drain for several seconds.

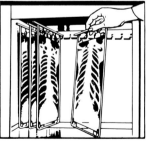

12 Dry Dry in dust-free area at room temperature or in suitable drying cabinet. Keep films well-separated. When dry, remove films from hangers and trim corners to remove clip marks. Insert in identified envelopes.

equal amount of time is required for the dissolved silver salts to diffuse out of the emulsion and for the gelatin to be "hardened" adequately.

If fixing time is longer than developing time, it may be convenient to have a fixer tank that is larger than the developer tank. When many films are being processed, the number of films in the fixer tank will build up relative to those in the developer as processing continues.

FIXATION PROCEDURE

Put the film into the solution and agitate it vigorously by moving it up and down several times; repeat periodically as recommended. This agitation will prevent stagnation of the solution in contact with the film so that fixation proceeds at a uniform rate. Follow the film manufacturer's recommendations for temperature and the time the film should be left in the fixer. This is usually at least twice the clearing time. Because the silver halide content of direct-exposure films is usually greater, their fixing time tends to be longer than for screen-type films. Keep in mind that the total fixing time is approximately twice the clearing time, and that films are sensitive to light until *after* fixation.

FIXER REPLENISHMENT

Unless the fixer solution is replenished, its activity diminishes with use. This results in longer times to fix films properly. Fixer replenishment maintains a minimum fixing time, thereby substantially increasing the fixing capacity of the processing system.

When using a fixer-replenishment system, remove the necessary amount of partially exhausted solution before adding replenisher. Because films and hangers carry about the same amount of liquid into the fixer tank as they carry out of it, the level of the fixer solution (unlike the developer) remains almost constant if little evaporation takes place.

WASHING

Films must be properly washed to remove the processing chemicals from the emulsion or the image will eventually discolor and fade. Proper washing requires an adequate supply of clean running water. It should flow so that both surfaces of each film will receive fresh water continuously. The hangers should be well-spaced in the tank and be completely immersed, including the top bar, so that the chemicals will also be removed from the tops of the frames.

The time required for adequate washing depends on water temperature, water quality, rate of water flow and turbulence, type of film, and somewhat, on the type of fixer. The temperature of the water should be close to that of the other solutions.

The water flow in the wash tank should be rapid enough to provide approximately eight complete changes of water per hour. Follow the film manufacturer's recommended washing times, which usually range from 5 to 30 minutes. Because its emulsions tend to be thicker, direct-exposure film requires longer washing. Washed and partially washed films absorb fixer chemicals from the contaminated wash water, as well as release them to the fresh water. Therefore, washing time should begin when the last film is immersed. To minimize contamination, put the films most recently introduced into the wash water from the fixer into the section of the tank nearest the outflow. Then, as more films are added, the older films, which contain less chemicals, can be moved upstream in a countercurrent direction–moving progressively closer to the inlet. This allows the films that are about to be removed for drying to be washed in the freshest water.

A washing method that uses a cascade system in which water flows through two or more small tanks is more efficient than one large tank. Preferably, water enters at the bottom of the second tank, flows past the film and out the top into the first tank. There it flows past the film most recently removed from the fixer and out through the drain in the bottom. The film should be allowed to drain for two to three seconds after being lifted from the wash water.

BIOLOGICAL GROWTH

A common problem with wash and processing solution tanks is the growth of slime deposits, particularly during seasons when the incoming water supply is warm. These slippery coatings are produced by bacteria, fungi, and to some extent, algae. Sources of contaminants originate from the air, personnel or the water supply. If not controlled, the deposits can cause both corrosion of metal surfaces and *artifacts* on radiographs. Control of these deposits requires continual housekeeping. Draining and scrubbing tanks with liquid household detergent at regular intervals is essential.

The use of filters in water supply lines and microbicides may also be helpful. Before using a microbicide, seek technical advice to determine that it is: (1) effective for the kind of growth present, (2) compatible with the process, and (3) in conformance with anti-pollution laws.

Information about biological growth control units that can be installed in a water supply line is available from manufacturers.

HYPO CLEARING AGENT

If the supply of wash water is limited, the capacity of the wash tanks insufficient, or there is not enough time to wash the film properly, use a *hypo clearing agent* or a *hypo eliminator* between the fixing and washing procedures. Treating the film with a hypo clearing agent permits a reduction in time and the quantity of water necessary for adequate washing.

WETTING AGENT

To help prevent water spots and drying marks on the radiograph and to reduce drying time, give the film a 30-second rinse in a *wetting agent* after removal from the wash water. The wetting agent reduces the surface tension of the water on the film, thereby preventing the formation of water droplets that create marks as they dry.

DRYING

This is the simplest step in processing, yet it is an important one. Improper drying may result in water marks or damage to the gelatin from excessive temperature. Drying temperatures should not exceed those recommended by the film manufacturer.

Wet, processed films are usually dried in cabinets fitted with heaters and fans to circulate the warmed air. Such dryers should be vented to the outside to prevent an excessive rise in temperature and humidity in the room.

Another type of dryer consists of a cabinet in which the moisture is withdrawn from the air by chemicals and the dehumidified air is recirculated over the film.

When dry, films should be removed promptly from the dryer to prevent them from becoming brittle. Corners should be trimmed to remove hanger clip marks. Films should be well-separated. If they come in contact with each other while drying, they will be damaged by drying marks or may stick together.

Copying Radiographs

COPYING

Duplicates of medical radiographs are often needed as teaching aids, for references, for inclusion with a patient's records or for other purposes. At one time, the production of such duplicates was a tedious undertaking requiring the use of solarization techniques. Direct-reversal duplicating films are available and high-quality duplicates of radiographs can be made quickly and conveniently.

To prevent blurring, the radiograph to be duplicated must be held in close contact with the emulsion side of the single-coated duplicating film during exposure. This may be accomplished by the use of a photographic printing frame or one of the commercially available mechanical or contact printers. The radiograph and film are arranged so that the exposing light passes through the radiograph to the emulsion of the duplicating film. Because it is a *reversal* film, increasing exposure reduces the density produced on a duplicating film. Therefore, a duplicate that is too low in density is corrected by decreasing the exposure. If the density of the copy is too high, the exposure should be increased to lower the density.

Duplicating film is designed for use with BLB (black light bulb) fluorescent lamps, which are rich in ultraviolet radiation. If poor results are obtained, contact your technical sales representative, try another brand of BLB, or do both. If other light sources, such as tungsten or daylight fluorescent lamps are used, the contrast of the duplicate will be incorrect.

SLIDES

It is possible to make 2 x 2-inch slides for screen projection from radiographs, or from other continuous-tone or line subjects, with direct-reversal films designed for use in 35 mm cameras. Some of these films can be processed in automatic processors.

SUBTRACTION

Sometimes a radiograph is cluttered with too much information. A lesion may be difficult to see because of the superimposed images of overlying or underlying structures. This problem frequently occurs in angiograms and may be lessened by the use of subtraction. Subtraction is a method of removing unwanted structures from a radiograph so that information of interest can be seen more easily. The procedure used is illustrated in **Figure F-1**.

In angiographic studies, subtraction can accentuate the pattern of blood vessels containing contrast media. This technique requires two radiographs, one (the base or scout radiograph) taken before and one (the angiogram) taken after the injection of contrast material. A reverse-tone subtraction mask is prepared by

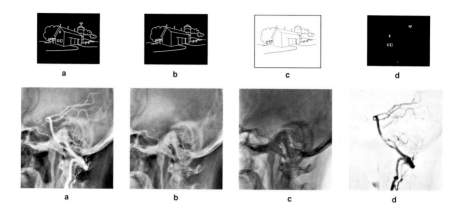

Figure F-1 Subtraction. **Top row.** **(a)** In this view of a rural scene, it is difficult to distinguish individual details in the drawing. **(b)** The part of the drawing in which we have no interest can be removed photographically. **(c)** By making a mask — a positive-reverse tone — of **b**, what was white in the original can be turned to black and vice versa. **(d)** If **a** is superimposed over **c**, the result shows that the unwanted portion of the scene has been canceled out, leaving only the individual details of interest. In other words, some structures have been subtracted to emphasize the presence of others. **Bottom Row.** **(a)** When we are interested in this specific anatomical detail and **(b)** other anatomical structures obscure this area, **(c)** the use of a subtraction mask can cancel out unwanted and interfering images. **(d)** The image shown here is the result of printing **c** over **a**.

making an exposure with the non-emulsion side of a sheet of subtraction masking film in contact with the scout radiograph. Cancellation of unwanted images is achieved by printing the mask in registration with the angiogram onto a subtraction print film. When the mask is placed over the angiogram, a uniform density is produced in all areas common to both films, leaving visible only those regions in which they differ, namely, where contrast material is present.

Information about films, equipment, and procedures for use in subtraction is available from film manufacturers.

Suggested Readings

Christensen's Physics of Diagnostic Radiology, Fourth Edition, Thomas S. Curry, III, James E. Dowdey, and Robert C. Murry, Jr., Lea & Febiger, 1990.

Concepts in Medical Radiographic Imaging—Circuitry, Exposure & Quality Control, Marianne Tortorici, W. B. Saunders Company, 1992.

Digital Imaging in Diagnostic Radiology, John D. Newell and Charles A. Kelsey, Editors, Churchill Livingstone, 1990.

Essentials of Radiology Physics, Charles A. Kelsey, Warren H. Green, Inc., 1985.

Film Processing in Medical Imaging, Arthur G. Haus, Editor, Medical Physics Publishing, 1993.

Mammographic Imaging—A Practical Guide, Valerie Fink Andolina, Shelly Lillé, and Kathleen M. Willison, J. B. Lippincott Company, 1992.

Mammography Quality Control—Radiologic Technologist's Manual, American College of Radiology, Committee on Quality Assurance in Mammography, 1992.

Medical Imaging Physics, Third Edition, William R. Hendee and E. Russell Ritenour, Mosby-Year Book Inc., 1992.

Physical Principles of Medical Imaging, Perry Sprawls, Jr., Aspen Publishers, Inc., 1987.

Physics of Medical Imaging: Recording System Measurements and Techniques, Arthur G. Haus, Editor, American Association of Physicists in Medicine, 1979.

Principles of Radiographic Imaging—An Art and a Science, Richard R. Carlton and Arlene McKenna Adler, Delmar Publishers, Inc. 1992.

Producing Quality Radiographs, Second Edition, Angeline M. Cullinan and John E. Cullinan, J. B. Lippincott Company, 1994.

Quality Control in Diagnostic Imaging, Joel E. Gray, Norlin T. Winkler, John Stears, and Eugene D. Frank, University Park Press, 1983.

Radiologic Science for Technologists—Physics, Biology, and Protection, Fifth Edition, Stewart C. Bushong, Mosby-Year Book Inc., 1993.

Screen Film Mammography—Imaging Considerations and Medical Physics Responsibilities, Gary T. Barnes and G. Donald Frey, Editors, Medical Physics Publishing, 1991.

References

1. National Electrical Manufacturers' Association (NEMA), Standard 1-8-1992.

2. Food and Drug Administration (FDA), 21 CFR Ch. 1 (4-1-92 Edition), 1020.30 (m) (1) Table 1.

3. "Technologic Improvements in Screen-Film Mammography," Arthur G. Haus, *Radiology*, Vol. 174, No. 3, pp. 628-637, March 1990.

4. "Minimizing Radiographic Blur," Perry Sprawls, Jr., Eastman Kodak Company, N-37, 1993.

5. "Screen Film Processing Systems for Medical Radiography: A Historical Review," Arthur G. Haus and John E. Cullinan, *RadioGraphics*, Vol. 9, No. 6, November 1989.

6. "Characteristics of KODAK Screen-Film Combinations for Conventional Medical Radiography," Arthur G. Haus and Robert E. Dickerson, Eastman Kodak Company, N-319, 1993.

7. "Automatic Film Processing in Medical Imaging: System Design Considerations," Arthur G. Haus, Thomas A. Batz, Robert E. Dickerson, Ronald F. Lillie, Kenneth W. Oemcke, and Jane D. Lanphear, Eastman Kodak Company, N-313, 1992.

8. "Screen-Film-Processing Systems and Quality Control in Mammography," Arthur G. Haus, Eastman Kodak Company, N-314, 1992.

9. "Processing of Mammographic Films: Technical and Clinical Considerations," László Tabár and Arthur G. Haus, *Radiology*, Vol. 173, No. 1, pp. 65-69, October 1989.

10. "Flood Replenishment: A new method of processor control," E. D. Frank, Joel E. Gray, and D. A. Wilken, *Radiologic Technology,* 52(3): 272-275, 1980.

11. The National Council on Radiation Protection and Measurement (NCRP) Report 99 on Quality Assurance, 1988.

12. American College of Radiology (ACR) *Mammography Quality Control Manual for Radiologic Technologists*, 1992.

13. "Evaluation of a clinical thermometer for measuring developer temperature in automatic film processor," W. B. Wilson, A. G. Haus, C. Nierman, R. Lillie, and T. A. Batz, *Medical Physics*, 20(3):823, 824, 1993.

14. "Some characteristics of the line spread function and modulation transfer function of medical radiographic films and screen-film systems," K. Rossmann and G. Lubberts, *Radiology* 1966:86, 235-241.

15. "Evaluation of Image Blur (Unsharpness) in Medical Imaging," Arthur G. Haus, Eastman Kodak Company, N-199, 1985.

16. *The Physical Aspects of Diagnostic Radiology*, Michel M. Ter-Pogossian, Hoeber Medical Division, Harper & Row, Publishers, Inc., 1967.

17. *Digital Imaging in Diagnostic Radiology*, John D. Newell, Jr. and Charles A. Kelsey, Churchill Livingston, 1990.

18. "Digital Radiography Using Storage Phosphors," Eastman Kodak Company, M3-430, 1992.

19. "Characteristics and Control of Contrast in CT," J. Ed Barnes, *RadioGraphics*, Vol. 12, No. 4, July 1992.

Glossary

absorption, x-ray: absorption (x-ray) describes the reduction in fluence as x rays traverse body tissues and emerge to expose an x-ray film.

aerial image: the pattern of x-ray fluence emerging from the body, incident on the image receptor; also referred to as the image in space.

afterglow: the tendency of a phosphor to continue to emit light after the x-ray exposure has stopped; also called phosphorescence.

ALARA: the acronym that represents the radiation protection philosophy that all radiation exposures should be kept "As Low As Reasonably Achievable."

alternating current (AC): electric current that reverses its polarity (direction of flow) and changes its magnitude at regularly recurring intervals.

amplitude: the magnitude of the deviation of a wave from its position of rest to either the crest or the trough.

anode: the component of an x-ray tube that contains the positively charged stationary or rotating target, which attracts negatively charged electrons from the cathode to produce x rays.

anti-foggant: a chemical added to film during emulsion manufacturing to keep the fog level to a minimum.

AP: anteroposterior, in a direction from the front to the back of a patient.

archiving: long-term storage of images, documents or digital data for subsequent retrieval.

artifact: any unwanted irregularity on the radiograph due to lint, dust, static electricity, film processing or improper storage or handling.

artifact, delay streaks: processing artifacts that run parallel to the direction in which film travels in a processor, visible on the leading edge of the film.

artifact, minus density: any unwanted artifact on film characterized by a white mark.

artifact, plus density: any unwanted artifact on film characterized by a black mark.

artifact, processor: any artifact arising from the automatic film processor.

attenuation, x-ray: see *absorption, x-ray*.

atomic number (Z): the number of protons in the nucleus of an atom.

automatic exposure control systems: automatic exposure control systems, often referred to as phototimers, automatically terminate the x-ray exposure, producing a predetermined level of exposure in the image.

automatic film processing: a processing method in which temperature, recirculation, and replenishment are automatically controlled as film is transported through processing solutions.

average gradient: the slope of the straight line joining corresponding points of specified densities on the characteristic curve. Used to indicate the contrast property of a film.

background radiation: radiation that occurs naturally in the environment.

backscatter: radiation that is scattered backward into the path of the original beam.

base plus fog: the optical density of the film base plus any additional density where no exposure has occurred.

beam quality: relative penetrating power of an x-ray beam. Increased beam quality refers to a more penetrating beam with a higher half-value layer (HVL).

blooming: the change in focal spot characteristics that occurs when a diagnostic x-ray tube is operated at decreased potential and increased tube current, compared with standard test conditions. NEMA Standard 1-8-1992.[1]

blur: a measure of the inability of all real systems to image the edge of an object with perfect fidelity. For example, blur causes the image of a 10-micrometer slit to be more than 10 micrometers wide.

Bucky mechanism: see *grid, moving.*

capacitor: a device for storing electricity.

cardboard film holder: a cardboard light-tight envelope used to hold direct-exposure x-ray film during a radiographic exposure.

cassette: a light-tight case, usually made of thin, low x-ray absorption plastic for holding x-ray film. One or two intensifying screens for the conversion of x rays to visible light photons, mounted inside the cassette in close contact with the film.

cathode: the negatively charged component of an x-ray tube that repels electrons towards the anode.

characteristic curve: a type of input-output response curve. In radiography, this curve expresses the change in optical density (output) with the change in exposure of x-ray film (input); also called H&D curve, D Log E curve or sensitometric curve.

cinefluorography: motion picture film recordings taken from the output phosphor of an image intensifier (fluoroscopy).

clearing agent: the agent in the fixer solution that dissolves the unexposed, undeveloped silver halide crystals, leaving the black metallic silver in the exposed and developed areas of the film more readily discernible; also called hypo.

collimator: a common term for a variable-aperture, beam-limiting device for restricting the field of x-ray photons in a beam to a desired shape and size.

cones: metal tubes of various shapes and sizes used to restrict the x-ray field.

contrast, film: a measure of a film's property to convert input changes in exposure (light or x-radiation) to output changes in optical density (film blackening).

contrast, radiographic: the difference in optical density (film blackening) between areas of interest in a radiograph. The combination of subject contrast and film contrast determines radiographic contrast.

contrast, subject: the ratio of x-ray photon fluences in the aerial image corresponding to different regions in the object being radiographed due to the effects of absorption.

contrast media: substances that are introduced into body tissue to enhance inherent x-ray absorption differences between body structures and the regions surrounding them. Contrast media may be radiopaque, such as barium, or radiolucent, such as air.

control limit: the maximum acceptable deviation or limit of film contrast, speed, and fog as plotted on a processor monitoring chart, used to monitor processor performance.

crossover: in dual-emulsion film, light from the front screen that penetrates the front emulsion layer and base, causing exposure and increased blur of the back emulsion.

cross-over assembly: part of an automatic film processor that is designed to move x-ray film from one section of a processor to another.

"crossover" procedure: a film processor quality control procedure used to correct differences in optical density introduced by a change in batches of film.

current: the flow of charged particles, for example, electrons.

densitometer: a device consisting of a light source, an aperture, and a light sensor, used to measure optical density.

D Log E curve: see *characteristic curve*.

density, optical: the degree of blackening of film after exposure and processing.

density, physical: the mass of a substance per unit volume. For example, grams/cm^3.

detail: a quality criterion corresponding to the ability of an imaging system to resolve small objects.

detective quantum efficiency (DQE): the square of the ratio of the output signal-to-noise ratio to the input signal-to-noise ratio. A measure of the efficiency with which photons are used for imaging.

developer: a chemical solution that converts the latent image on film to a visible image.

digital: a numerical representation of discrete values, typically used by computers.

digital radiography: an image acquisition process that produces radiographic images in digital form.

distortion: an inaccurately shaped shadow or aerial image of an object that occurs whenever an object is not parallel to the image receptor. Distortion also occurs by angulation of the x-ray tube with respect to the image receptor.

D-Max: see *maximum density*.

dose: a measure of the energy absorbed per unit mass. 1 gray equals 100 rads.

dose, average glandular: generally used in breast dosimetry. Determined from values of entrance exposure in air, the x-ray beam quality (half-value layer), and compressed breast thickness. Average glandular dose is the energy deposited per unit mass of glandular tissue (by far the most radiosensitive tissue in the breast) averaged over all the glandular tissue in the breast; also called mean glandular dose.

dose rate, absorbed: rads per minute received at a point of interest.

electromagnetic spectrum: the range of all electromagnetic radiations according to their energy.

electron: a minute negatively charged particle that revolves around the positively charged nucleus in assigned orbits or shells.

element: a substance that is composed exclusively of atoms having the same atomic number, which cannot be separated into simpler substances by ordinary chemical means.

emulsion, film: a mixture of gelatin and silver halide crystals (in suspension) where latent image formation takes place.

exposure: a measure of the amount of ionization produced in air by an x-ray beam, measured in mR (milliroentgens) or R (Roentgens).

exposure rate: Roentgens per minute measured at a point of interest.

extra-focal radiation: x-radiation produced from electron interaction with metal other than the focal spot of the x-ray tube; also called off-focus radiation.

FFD: see *focal-film distance.*

FOD: see *focal-object distance.*

film, direct-exposure: silver halide film primarily sensitive to the direct action of x rays but having low sensitivity to light from screen fluorescence.

film speed: the sensitivity of film emulsion to x-ray or light exposure.

film, x-ray: silver halide film that is primarily sensitized to the spectrum of light emitted by fluorescent intensifying screens.

filtration, added: a material or device inserted between the x-ray tube and the patient to preferentially absorb lower energy photons from an x-ray beam.

filtration, inherent: the effect of all components (such as the glass wall of a tube) that filter the x-ray beam from its production in the target until it emerges from the x-ray tube.

filtration, total: the equivalent amount of filtering material (usually stated in millimeters of aluminum) between the focal spot and the object being radiographed; also the sum of the added and inherent filtration.

fixer: a chemical solution that both removes the unexposed and undeveloped silver halide crystals from the coated film emulsion and hardens the gelatin.

flooded replenishment: a technique used in low-volume processing that adjusts replenishment pumps in an automatic film processor to automatically add a predetermined amount of developer and fixer replenisher on a timed cycle to maintain the chemical activity of the processor; also called flood replenishment.

fluence: in electromagnetic imaging, the number of photons per unit area.

fluorescence: the property of a phosphor to emit light in the visible region of the electromagnetic spectrum as a result of absorbing higher energy radiation, such as x rays.

focal distance, grid: the distance from the point of convergence or focal point of x rays to a focused grid.

focal-film distance (FFD): the distance from the anode target (focus) of an x-ray tube to the radiographic film; also referred to as the target-film distance (TFD) or the source-image receptor distance (SID).

focal-object distance (FOD): the distance from the focal spot or target of an x-ray tube to the object being radiographed; also called the target-object distance (TOD) or the source-object distance (SOD).

focal range: a range of distances, specified by grid manufacturers, within which a focused grid can be satisfactorily used.

focal spot, actual: the primary source of x rays produced at the location where the anode of an x-ray tube intercepts the electron beam. NEMA Standard 1-8-92.[1]

focal track: the area that electrons strike on a rotating anode.

focusing cup: the part of an x-ray tube's cathode that holds the tungsten filaments and shapes the electron stream to a small region on the target.

fog: an unwanted exposure to the film emulsion from light, radiation, heat or chemicals; also refers to the optical density on a processed radiograph arising from this exposure.

Fourier transform: a mathematical process used to convert the line spread function (LSF) to the modulation transfer function (MTF).

gamma: the slope of the straight-line portion of the characteristic curve that is related to film contrast.

gelatin: the material made from animal tissue in which silver halide crystals are suspended to make an emulsion.

generator: a machine that converts AC electrical power into a waveform suitable for the production of x rays.

gradient: the slope of the tangent to the characteristic curve at a given density.

graininess: the appearance of optical density fluctuations on film, caused by the random inhomogeneous distribution of silver grains as they are unevenly coated in the emulsion.

granularity: the microdensitometric measurement of the graininess fluctuations in an emulsion.

gray (Gy): A unit of absorbed dose or energy deposited in tissue. 1 gray equals 100 rad.

gray scale: the range of optical densities present in an image.

grid: a device composed of parallel or slanted lead strips and radiolucent spacer material, used to reduce scattered radiation.

grid cutoff: a decrease in x-ray fluence caused by misalignment between the lead strips of a grid and the diverging primary beam.

grid ratio: the relationship of the height of the lead strips in a grid to the width of its radiolucent spacers.

grid, crosshatch: a grid consisting of two linear grids, one perpendicular to and on top of the other, used to reduce scattered radiation; also referred to as a crisscrossed grid.

grid, focused: a grid used to reduce scattered radiation, in which lead strips are progressively tilted bilaterally to align with the diverging x rays emanating from the focal spot.

grid, moving: a device comprised of a stationary grid and a mechanism for moving it that blurs the image of the grid lines, making them indistinguishable on the radiographic film; also referred to as a Bucky mechanism.

grid, parallel: a device used to reduce scattered radiation with lead strips that are parallel; also called an unfocused grid.

H & D curve: see *characteristic curve*.

halation: a double image or "halo" effect that occurs when some of the exposing light penetrates the film emulsion and is reflected back by the film support.

half-value layer (HVL): the thickness of a given material required to reduce x-ray beam fluence to one-half of its original (unattenuated) value.

heel effect: the variation in fluence across the x-ray beam associated with the angle of the x-ray target.

hertz (Hz): the unit used to measure temporal (time) frequency. One hertz is equivalent to one cycle per second.

hypo: see *clearing agent*.

image blur: see *blur*.

image in space: see *aerial image*.

image processing: any operation performed to enhance or clarify an image as an aid in diagnosis.

image quality, radiographic: a description or quantitative measure of the excellence of an image with respect to contrast, blur, noise, and artifacts.

image receptor: the x-ray detection material (for example, intensifying screen(s) with radiographic film) on which a latent image corresponding to the aerial image is formed.

image, latent: the invisible changes that occur in an unprocessed image receptor and which arise from x-ray exposure.

instantaneous load: the highest kVp and mAs values that can be used for a given length of time for a single exposure with a specific x-ray tube.

intrinsic efficiency: the ratio of light energy generated in a phosphor crystal to the x-ray energy absorbed by the crystal; also called phosphor conversion efficiency.

inverse square law: the relationship between distance and radiation fluence in which the exposure varies inversely as the square of the distance from the source.

ionization chamber: a device that produces an electric current when exposed to ionizing radiation.

keV: thousand electron volts.

kilo: a prefix, used with a unit of measure, indicating that the unit should be multiplied by one thousand. For example, one kilovolt (kV) is equivalent to one thousand volts.

kilovoltage, peak (kVp): the maximum potential difference between anode and cathode in an x-ray tube.

kVp: see *kilovoltage, peak*.

latitude, exposure: a measure of the tolerance allowed in the choice of exposure values required to produce the desired density range.

latitude, film: the capability of a film emulsion to record a wide range of exposures, resulting in the film having a lower inherent contrast. Wide-latitude film is often used for chest radiography.

line-focus principle: the phenomenon that results in the difference between the size and shape of the actual focal spot and the effective focal spot, caused by the angle of the target of an x-ray tube.

line spread function (LSF): spatial distribution of optical density in the slit image of an x-ray beam.

maximum density: the highest optical density that would be obtained if all the silver halide grains on a film were developed; also referred to as saturation density or D-Max.

MeV: million electron volts.

milli: a prefix, used with a unit of measure, indicating that the unit should be multiplied by one one-thousandth. For example, one millisecond (ms) equals one one-thousandth of a second.

milliamperage (mA): a measure of the number of electrons flowing per second; also called milliamperes.

milliampere-seconds (mAs): the product of the factors milliamperes and time, used to calculate changes in exposure, mAs = mA x time (sec.).

modulation transfer function (MTF): a graphic representation of the resolution capability of an imaging system or component.

monochromatic radiation: a beam of ionizing radiation in which all the photons are essentially of equal energy.

mottle, quantum: a type of radiographic mottle due to the statistical variation in the number of photons incident on any given area of the image receptor.

mottle, screen: an image imperfection resulting from the structural composition of the fluorescent screen; also known as structure mottle.

National Electrical Manufacturers' Association (NEMA): an organization of manufacturers active in standardization.

neutrons: an atomic particle with no charge that is similar in mass to the proton, and is a constituent of all atomic nuclei except that of hydrogen.

noise: any undesired variation of input or output signal that interferes with the detection of the desired signal.

nucleus: the positively charged central portion of an atom, which contains protons and neutrons.

object-film distance (OFD): the distance from the object to the film.

OFD: see *object-film distance.*

off-focus radiation: see *extra-focal radiation.*

overcoat: a very thin layer of clear gelatin in film, usually coated on top of the emulsion layer to protect it from abrasion and provide important surface properties.

OID: object-image receptor distance.

PA: posteroanterior, in a direction from the back to the front of a patient.

parallax effect: the impression of a change in position of an object as seen on dual-emulsion film when a tube-angled technique is used.

phantom: a test object that simulates the x-ray absorption of various structures within the body.

phosphor conversion efficiency: see *intrinsic efficiency.*

phosphorescence: the ability of phosphor to emit light as a result of the previous absorption of higher energy radiation, such as x rays; see *afterglow.*

photomultiplier: an electronic device that converts varying light intensities (from a storage phosphor screen) into varying electrical signals.

photon: a bundle of electromagnetic energy.

phototimer: an electronic timing device that automatically measures and terminates the x-ray exposure to achieve a preselected density on a radiograph.

pixel: an abbreviation for *pic*ture *el*ement.

positive beam limitation (PBL) device: a beam-limiting device that automatically limits the x-ray beam to the size of the image receptor.

Potter-Bucky diaphragm: a device comprised of a stationary grid and a mechanism for moving it that blurs the image of the grid's lines and makes them indistinguishable on radiographic film; also referred to as a Bucky mechanism.

primary beam: the beam of x rays emitted from the focal spot that have not been scattered.

primary beam leak: the unattenuated portion of the x-ray beam that strikes the table or cassette causing image undercutting.

processing cycle: the amount of time required for the leading edge of the film to enter and the trailing edge to exit an automated processor; also called drop time.

processor, automatic film: a machine that transports film through developing, fixing, washing, and drying sections to produce a finished radiograph.

processor monitoring chart: a chart used to record and monitor performance of a film processor in a quality control program.

proton: an elementary particle in the atomic nucleus that has a positive charge equal to that of the electron but with much greater mass.

quantum: a packet or bundle of electromagnetic energy.

quantum theory: the theory that electromagnetic energy is transferred in discrete quanta or photons.

rad: a unit of radiation dose. 1 gray equals 100 rads.

radiograph: an image captured on film (or other hard copy media) that is created as a result of differential absorption of radiation by objects in the x-ray beam.

radiolucent: relatively permeable to x rays or gamma rays.

radiopaque: relatively impermeable to x rays or other forms of radiation.

reciprocity law: a law stating that the optical density of a radiograph will be the same if the milliampere-seconds (mAs) is constant, regardless of mA.

rectification: the conversion of an alternating current to a direct current.

rectifier: an electrical device used to convert alternating current to direct current, permitting electric current to flow in one direction only.

replenishment: manually or automatically adding fresh chemicals to developer and fixer solutions to maintain proper chemical activity, stability, and liquid levels.

replenishment rate: the amount of replenisher chemicals added to the developer and fixer solutions based on film type, film size, and usage rate (number of sheets of film processed in 24 hrs).

resolution: the ability of an imaging system to visually distinguish closely spaced lines.

Roentgen (R): a unit of radiation exposure measured in air.

safelight: a device containing a low-wattage light bulb and filter that produces visible light to which film is relatively insensitive, while still allowing one to see in the darkroom.

saturation density: see *maximum density*.

scatter: any radiation from sources other than the primary x-ray beam.

screen conversion efficiency: the ratio of the light energy emitted by an intensifying screen to the x-ray energy absorbed by the screen.

screen-film contact: the close proximity of the intensifying screen to the film emulsion that is necessary to minimize image blur.

screen speed: a measure of the relative light output of various intensifying screens for a given x-ray exposure.

sensitometer: a device that exposes film to a controlled, stepped set of light exposures. It is used to evaluate a film's response to exposure.

SID: source-image receptor distance.

signal: an electronic representation of information.

silver halide: a compound produced by mixing a solution of silver nitrate with a solution of potassium halide. Used in photographic emulsions because of its sensitivity to light and other forms of radiation.

silver recovery: any method in which a recovery unit removes silver from the fixer effluent.

slit camera: a device used in the measurement of the focal spot of an x-ray tube.

SOD: source-object distance.

source-image receptor distance (SID): see *focal-film distance.*

source-object distance (SOD): see *focal-object distance.*

spatial distribution: a distribution of particles, such as photons, silver grains or water droplets, as a function of space or distance.

spectrum (x-ray): the distribution of x-ray photons (relative number and energy) in an x-ray beam.

SSD: source-skin distance.

speed: a measure of the exposure needed to produce a given density on film.

stepped-wedge: a device with graduated thicknesses that is used to demonstrate or test various degrees of x-ray penetration; also known as a step-wedge.

subtraction: a radiographic, photographic or digital electronic technique in which unwanted information can be subtracted from images to enhance the visibility of the desired information. Subtraction is especially useful in angiography.

target (x-ray tube): the part of the anode in an x-ray tube towards which electrons from the cathode are focused and attracted and where they interact to produce x-radiation.

target-film distance (TFD): see *focal-film distance*.

target-object distance (TOD): see *focal-object distance*.

thermionic emission: the escape of electrons from the heated filament in the cathode of an x-ray tube.

time-temperature processing: a technique used in manual processing that involves adjusting development time and developer temperature to produce optimum optical density and image quality for a given exposure.

tube rating charts: information provided in chart form by the manufacturer to prevent damage to an x-ray tube from excessive heat.

undercutting: localized scattered radiation that is generated when a portion of the x-ray beam extends beyond the edge of the part being radiographed (primary beam leak).

variable-aperture, beam-limiting device: see *collimator*.

viewbox: a device that provides a uniform field of white light for viewing the radiographic image.

viewing station: an electronic device for the display of text and medical images in digital format.

voxel: abbreviation for *vo*lume *el*ement, referring to the location in a patient represented by a pixel.

wave: a variation or disturbance that transfers energy progressively from point to point in a medium.

workstation: an electronic device for the display, manipulation, and evaluation of text and digital images.

Index

Figures are represented by *f* following their page number.

Figures are represented by *f* following their page number.

Figures are represented by *f* following their page number.